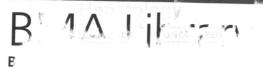
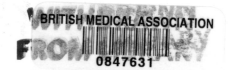

Hepatology
CLINICAL CASES UNCOVERED

Kathryn Nash
MA, PhD, MRCP
Consultant Hepatologist
Southampton General Hospital
Southampton, UK

Indra Neil Guha
MBBS, MRCP, PhD
Clinical Associate Professor in Hepatology
University of Nottingham
Nottingham, UK

WILEY-BLACKWELL
A John Wiley & Sons, Ltd., Publication

This edition first published 2011, © 2011 by Kathryn Nash and Indra Neil Guha

Blackwell Publishing was acquired by John Wiley & Sons in February 2007. Blackwell's publishing program has been merged with Wiley's global Scientific, Technical and Medical business to form Wiley-Blackwell.

Registered office: John Wiley & Sons Ltd, The Atrium, Southern Gate, Chichester, West Sussex, PO19 8SQ, UK

Editorial offices: 9600 Garsington Road, Oxford, OX4 2DQ, UK
The Atrium, Southern Gate, Chichester, West Sussex, PO19 8SQ, UK
111 River Street, Hoboken, NJ 07030-5774, USA

For details of our global editorial offices, for customer services and for information about how to apply for permission to reuse the copyright material in this book please see our website at www.wiley.com/wiley-blackwell

Library of Congress Cataloging-in-Publication Data
Nash, Kathryn.
    Hepatology : clinical cases uncovered / Kathryn Nash, Indra Neil Guha.
        p. ; cm.
    Includes bibliographical references and index.
    ISBN 978-1-4443-3246-9 (pbk. : alk. paper)
1. Liver–Diseases–Case studies.   I. Guha, Indra Neil.   II. Title.
    [DNLM: 1. Liver Diseases–Case Reports.   2. Liver Diseases–Problems and Exercises.   WI 18.2]
    RC845.N36 2011
    616.3'62–dc22
                                    2010047396

ISBN: 9781444332469

A catalogue record for this book is available from the British Library

Set in 9/12 pt Minion by Toppan Best-set Premedia Limited

Printed and bound in Malaysia by Vivar Printing Sdn Bhd

1   2011

Contents

Preface

Welcome to *Clinical Cases Uncovered: Hepatology*. We have tried to create a book that is informative, interesting and relevant to everyday clinical practice. The strength of this book, like others in the series, is that we use real clinical cases to illustrate liver disease, highlighting the anatomical, physiological and pathological basis behind each case. We hope the reader will appreciate some of the nuances of the clinical management of liver disease that are often not documented in traditional textbooks but which we have tried to highlight through these cases. The cases themselves come directly from our personal clinical practice from a variety of settings including busy district general hospitals, teaching hospitals and liver transplant centres. We are grateful to our previous teachers and mentors who have inspired us and hope that we can share their enthusiasm and wisdom with you.

Hepatology is becoming an increasingly important part of everyday clinical practice. The incidence of liver disease has risen at an exponential rate over the last 30 years, due to a mixture of alcohol, obesity and viral hepatitis. Most general medicine takes encounter patients with liver disease, and every general practice will care for several such patients.

Hepatology is not a 'dark art', nor is it solely a postgraduate topic, but rather it is a fascinating subject that affects many other body systems including the heart, lungs, kidneys and brain. The principles of successful management of patients with acute liver disease are common to the management of any acutely unwell patient.

We have thoroughly enjoyed writing this book and hope that not only will it increase your knowledge and confidence in dealing with liver disease, but that it will also be a highly stimulating journey.

Kathryn Nash
Neil Guha

Acknowledgements

We would like to thank our colleagues in Southampton and Nottingham: Dr Guru Aithal, Dr Steven Ryder, Dr Martin James, Dr Mark Wright and Dr Nick Sheron for their support. We are particularly indebted to Dr Martin James for help in obtaining images, Dr Adrian Bateman for the pathology photographs and Mr Christopher Watson for images, the initial idea and encouragement throughout.

Some figures in this book are taken from: Ellis H. & Watson C. (2008). *Clinical Cases Uncovered: Surgery*. Wiley-Blackwell, Oxford.

We would like to give our special thanks to both our families for their enduring support and love and for everything they did behind the scenes that allowed us the time to write this book.

 # How to use this book

Clinical Cases Uncovered (CCU) books are carefully designed to help supplement your clinical experience and assist with refreshing your memory when revising. Each book is divided into three sections: Part 1, Basics; Part 2, Cases; and Part 3, Self-assessment.

Part 1 gives you a quick reminder of the basic science, history and examination, and key diagnoses in the area. Part 2 contains many of the clinical presentations you would expect to see on the wards or to crop up in exams, with questions and answers leading you through each case. New information, such as test results, is revealed as events unfold and each case concludes with a handy case summary explaining the key points. Part 3 allows you to test your learning with several question styles (MCQs, EMQs and SAQs), each with a strong clinical focus.

Whether reading individually or working as part of a group, we hope you will enjoy using your CCU book. If you have any recommendations on how we could improve the series, please do let us know by contacting us at: medicalstudent@wiley.co.uk.

Disclaimer
CCU patients are designed to reflect real life, with their own reports of symptoms and concerns. Please note that all names used are entirely fictitious and any similarity to patients, alive or dead, is coincidental.

Normal values

Alanine aminotransferase (ALT)	10–40 iU/L	Haemoglobin (Hb)	110–150 g/dL (female) 130–170 g/dL (male)
Albumin	35–48 g/L	HbA_{1c}	4–6.5%
Alkaline phosphatase (ALP)	35–105 iU/L	Immunoglobulin G	6–16 g/L
α_1-antitrypsin level	1.1–2.2 g/L	INR	0.8–1.2
α-fetoprotein (AFP)	0–10 iU/mL	Mean corpuscular volume (MCV)	80–100 fL
Bilirubin	0–20 μmol/L		
C-reactive protein (CRP)	0–7.5 mg/L	Neutrophils	$2.0–7.5 \times 10^9$/L
Cholesterol (HDL)	≥1 mmol/L	Platelets (Plt)	$150–400 \times 10^9$/L
Cholesterol : HDL ratio	≤4	Potassium	3.5–5.0 mmol/L
Cholesterol (total)	≤5.0 mmol/L	Prothrombin time (PT)	10–14 seconds
Creatinine	80–115 μmol/L	Sodium	136–144 mmol/L
Creatinine kinase (CK)	38–174 iU/L	Triglycerides	0.45–1.8 mmol/L
Ferritin	23.9–336 μg/L	Urea	2.9–7.1 mmol/L
γ-glutamyl transferase	11–50 iU/L	White blood cells (WBC)	$4–11 \times 10^9$/L
Glucose	4.0–6.0 mmol/L		

List of abbreviations

AFLP	acute fatty liver of pregnancy		5-HIAA	5-hydroxyindoleacetic acid
AFP	alpha-fetoprotein		HIV	human immunodeficiency virus
ALP	alkaline phosphatase		5-HT	5-hydroxytryptamine
ALT	alanine aminotransferase		ICP	intrahepatic cholestasis of pregnancy
AMA	antimitochondrial antibody		Ig	immunoglobulin
ANA	antinuclear antibody		INR	international normalised ratio
AST	aspartate aminotransferase		IV	intravenous
ATP	adenosine triphosphate		IVC	inferior vena cava
BMI	body mass index		LDL	low density lipoprotein
BP	blood pressure		LFT	liver function test
BRIC	benign recurrent intrahepatic cholestasis		LVP	large volume paracentesis
CCK	cholecystokinin		MR	magnetic resonance
CEA	carcinoembryonic antigen		MRCP	magnetic resonance cholangiopancreatography
CK	creatinine kinase			
CMV	cytomegalovirus		MRI	magnetic resonance imaging
CRP	C-reactive protein		NAFLD	non-alcoholic fatty liver disease
CT	computed tomography		NAPQI	N-acetyl-p-benzoquionimine
CVP	central venous pressure		NASH	non-alcoholic steatohepatitis
CXR	chest X-ray		NBM	nil by mouth
DEXA	dual energy X-ray absorptiometry		NSAIDs	non-steroidal anti-inflammatory drugs
DNA	deoxyribonucleic acid		PBC	primary biliary cirrhosis
EBV	Epstein–Barr virus		PET	positron emission tomography
ECG	electrocardiogram		PIII NP	serum type III procollagen peptide
ERCP	endoscopic retrograde cholangiopancreatography		Plt	platelets
			PSC	primary sclerosing cholangitis
ESR	erythrocyte sedimentation rate		PT	prothombin time
EUS	endoscopic ultrasound		PTC	percutaneous transhepatic cholangiography
^{18}FDG	fluorodeoxyglucose		RFA	radiofrequency ablation
γ-GT	gamma glutamyl transferase		SAAG	serum albumin–ascites albumin gradient
G6PD	glucose-6-phosphate dehydrogenase		SBP	spontaneous bacterial peritonitis
GI	gastrointestinal		STEMI	ST segment elevation myocardial infarction
GP	general practitioner		TB	tuberculosis
HAART	highly active antiretroviral therapy		TIPS	transjugular intrahepatic portosystemic shunt
Hb	haemoglobin			
HBV	hepatitis B virus		TNF-α	tumour necrosis factor alpha
HCC	hepatocellular carcinoma		UDP	uridine diphosphate
HDL	high density lipoprotein		VLDL	very low density lipoprotein
HDV	hepatitis D virus		WBC	white blood cells

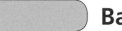

Basic science

Anatomy

The liver is the largest solid organ in the body weighing approximately 1600 g in men and 1400 g in women. It lies in the right upper quadrant of the abdomen under the rib cage with its upper border between the fifth and sixth ribs and its lower border along the right costal margin where it can sometimes be palpated on inspiration in healthy subjects (Fig. A).

Embryological development of the liver

To understand the anatomy and vascular relationships of the adult liver it is first necessary to review its development.

Hepatic parenchyma

The primitive liver develops in the 3-week-old embryo as an outgrowth from the distal ventral wall of the foregut. This liver bud, or hepatic diverticulum, proliferates into solid cords of endodermal cells which invade the mesenchyme of the nearby septum transversum. A series of branching and anastomosing plates spread between the umbilical and vitelline veins forming a close relationship, which eventually develops into the hepatocytes and sinusoids of the mature liver parenchyma.

Biliary system

The hepatic diverticulum divides, the large cranial part forming the hepatic parenchyma and the smaller caudal part forming an epithelial cord extending from the hepatic parenchyma to the foregut, the eventual duodenum. This solid cord becomes vacuolated forming a lumen first in the common bile duct and then in the hepatic duct, cystic duct and gallbladder. The intrahepatic ducts begin to form from the hepatocytes in direct contact with the mesenchyme at week 9–10. Epithelial and mesenchymal resorption and remodelling occurs, resulting in a network of biliary tubules. Disturbance of this remodelling process is responsible for a number of disorders including congenital hepatic fibrosis, Caroli's disease and polycystic liver disease.

Venous system

The hepatic venous system develops from four veins: two umbilical veins carrying oxygenated blood from the placenta, and two vitelline veins draining into the sinus venosus (Fig. B(a)). By week 7 the definitive fetal circulation is formed (Fig. B(b)):

• The right umbilical vein and the cranial portion of the left umbilical vein regress and disappear.
• The remainder of the left umbilical vein persists providing the principal source of placental blood.
• A new vessel, the ductus venosus, develops forming a bypass channel connecting the umbilical vein to the inferior vena cava.
• The upper anastomoses of the vitelline veins develop into a single portal vein with left and right branches.
• The distal vitelline veins form the superior mesenteric and splenic veins.
• At birth, blood flow ceases in the umbilical vein, the ductus venosus closes and the portal vein takes over the venous blood supply to the liver. The obliterated segment of the umbilical vein between the umbilicus and the left portal vein branch regresses to form the ligamentum teres, and the ductus venosus becomes a fibrous cord, the ligamentum venosum, running in the right lobe (Fig. B(c)).

Gross anatomy

The liver is divided into two uneven lobes, the right and left, by the falciform ligament, which is a remnant of the embryonic umbilical vein. These 'anatomical lobes' have no functional significance. The right lobe is larger than the left and contains the quadrate and caudate lobes (Fig. C(a) and(b)). Between the quadrate and caudate lobes is the porta hepatitis or liver hilum. Here the portal vein

Hepatology: Clinical Cases Uncovered, 1st edition. © Kathryn Nash and Indra Neil Guha. Published 2011 by Blackwell Publishing Ltd.

and hepatic artery enter and the bile ducts leave the liver. In some individuals there is a downward protrusion of the anterior edge of the right lobe of the liver known as Riedel's lobe*. It may extend into the right iliac fossa and be palpable. It is considered as a normal variant.

Apart from an area on its posterior surface, the bare area, the liver is covered by a fibrous capsule, Glisson's capsule.[†] The bare area lies in direct contact with the diaphragm and is surrounded by reflections of peritoneum. The falciform ligament attaches the liver to the diaphragm and anterior abdominal wall. Its anterior portion, the round ligament (ligamentum teres), connects the left branch of the portal vein to the umbilicus. It contains small vestigial veins that can reopen and become varicose if intrahepatic portal venous hypertension develops.

Liver vasculature and functional anatomy

The liver receives about a quarter of the resting cardiac output via a dual blood supply:

• The portal vein provides approximately 75% of hepatic blood flow. It is formed by the union of the superior mesenteric and splenic veins and drains venous blood from most of the digestive tract, spleen, pancreas and gallbladder (Fig. D).

• The hepatic artery, the second major branch of the coeliac axis, provides the remaining 25% of hepatic blood flow, but 50% of the oxygen supply. The hepatic arteries give rise to branches that supply the biliary epithelium, thus obstruction to arterial flow can result in the development of an ischaemic cholangitis.

The distribution of the hepatic blood supply and biliary drainage divides the liver functionally into two roughly equal 'physiological lobes'. The line of demarcation between right and left vascular inflow passes along

Figure A The position of the liver in health.

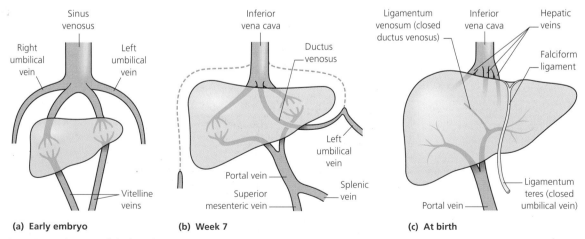

(a) Early embryo   **(b) Week 7**   **(c) At birth**

Figure B Development of the hepatic venous system.

---

*Bernhard Moritz Carl Ludwig Riedel (1846–1916), German surgeon.

[†]Francis Glisson (*c.* 1599–1677), British physician and anatomist, and Regius Professor of Physics, Cambridge.

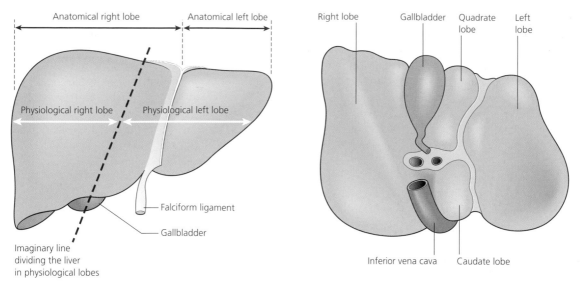

(a) Anterior view

(b) Inferior view

Figure C Gross anatomy of the liver.

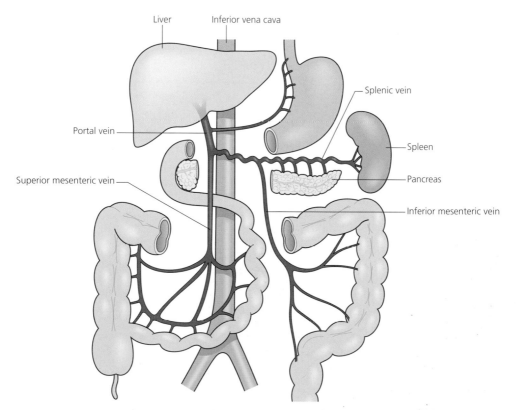

Figure D Anatomy of the portal vein.

a plane joining the tip of the gallbladder to the groove of the inferior vena cava (see Fig. C(a)). The understanding of this vascular anatomy and the recognition of true right and left lobes is of major importance in radiologically staging hepatic tumours and in surgical resection of the liver.

The liver is drained by three major veins, the right, middle and left hepatic veins. As they emerge from the posterior surface of the liver the left and middle veins usually join, forming a common trunk that drains alongside the right hepatic vein into the inferior vena cava just before it passes through the diaphragm. In addition to the main hepatic veins, small inferior veins drain the posterior segment of the right lobe and the caudate lobe directly into the vena cava. This arrangement protects the caudate lobe from injury and allows it to hypertrophy if the main hepatic veins are occluded (Budd–Chiari syndrome).

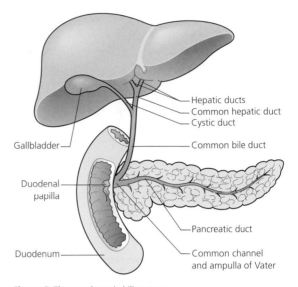

Figure E The extrahepatic biliary tree.

Biliary drainage

Within the hepatic parenchyma bile canaliculi form an anastomosing network between the hepatocytes. They join near the portal tracts and form progressively larger ducts, eventually creating right and left hepatic ducts which leave the right and left liver lobes, respectively. The hepatic ducts meet at the porta hepatis and unite, forming the common hepatic duct. The gallbladder lies under the right lobe of the liver where it stores and concentrates bile. It is drained by the cystic duct, which joins the common hepatic duct to form the common bile duct. The common bile duct runs behind the first part of the duodenum in the groove on the back of the head of the pancreas and enters the second part of the duodenum, usually joining the main pancreatic duct to form a common channel, the ampulla of Vater (Fig. E). The lower end of the common bile duct contains the muscular sphincter of Oddi which prevents bile entering the duodenum in the fasting state. In about 30% of individuals, the bile duct and pancreatic duct open separately into the duodenum.

Intrahepatic organisation

The hepatic artery and portal vein enter the porta hepatitis within a sheath of connective tissue, the gastroduodenal ligament, which also contains bile duct branches as they leave the liver. The vessels run parallel and branch in all directions eventually emptying into the hepatic sinusoids. Blood passes from the portal tract via the hepatic sinusoids to the terminal vein (central vein). The hepatic veins run in the opposite direction to the portal tract with terminal hepatic venules collecting blood from the sinusoids and forming larger channels leading to the main hepatic veins.

Two models have been proposed for the functional unit of the liver (Figs F and G):

1 The classic lobule (Fig. F) is a hexagonal structure organised around a central venule, a tributary of the hepatic vein, with the portal tracts forming the corners of the hexagon. This model is convenient for describing centrilobular or perilobular structural alterations occurring around the hepatic venule or portal tracts, respectively, but it is not an isolated functional unit.

2 The liver acinus (Fig. G) more accurately describes the functional unit of the liver and describes the hepatic parenchyma in zones:

  • Hepatocytes in zone 1 are closest to the portal triad; they receive the richest supply of oxygen and nutrients but are more likely to be damaged by drugs and toxins as they are exposed to higher concentrations of these.

  • Zone 3 hepatocytes are near the central vein and have a relatively poor oxygen supply and are therefore particularly susceptible to hypoxic damage.

Tissues of the liver
Hepatocytes

Eighty to 85% of the liver volume is made up of hepatocytes – polyhedral-shaped, polarised epithelial cells. The

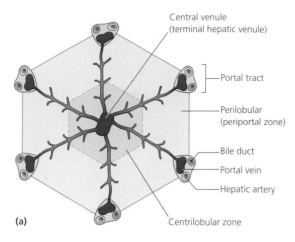

(a)

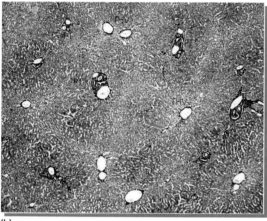

(b)

Figure F Proposed models for the functional unit of the liver. (a) Classic lobule. (b) Normal liver showing the spatial relationship between the portal tracts (PT) and terminal hepatic venules (THV). (Reticulin stain.)

cells are arranged in plates with the basolateral surface projecting into the perisinusoidal space of Disse where they are in direct contact with cell-free blood.

Cholangiocytes

The bile ducts are composed of epithelial cells, called cholangiocytes. The cells lining the small interlobular ducts are cuboidal, whereas those of the larger bile ducts are columnar, mucus-secreting cells.

Cells of the sinusoid

The vascular sinusoids are lined by endothelial cells that contain numerous fenestrae allowing free passage of solutes into the space of Disse that lies between the sinu-soidal endothelial cells and the hepatocytes (Fig. H). This space of Disse contains perisinusoidal cells, the hepatic stellate cells also known as Ito cells. These are multifunctional cells involved in fat and vitamin storage and with the potential to transform into fibroblasts, which are a major source of extracellular matrix in the normal and diseased liver. Kupffer cells float freely in the lumen of the sinusoids. They are members of the mononuclear phagocytic system and are responsible for the clearance of particles, injured red cells and toxins. Liver-associated lymphocytes can be recruited from the peripheral blood to the liver sinusoids where they mature and acquire natural and lymphokine-activated cell activity.

Lymphatics

Hepatic lymph is formed by drainage of the perisinusoidal space of Disse into lymphatic plexuses of the portal tract. The lymphatic plexuses progressively enlarge as they follow the portal vessels to the portal hepatitis, and the majority drain into hepatic lymph nodes at the liver hilum. Other drainage routes occur via the falciform ligament and epigastric vessels to the parasternal nodes, from the liver surface to the left gastric nodes and from the bare area to the posterior mediastinal nodes.

Nerve supply

Nerve plexuses around the hepatic artery and portal vein provide parasympathetic fibres from the vagus nerve and sympathetic fibres from the coeliac ganglia.

Physiology
Bile formation and excretion

Bile secretion is an important exocrine function of the liver. Bile is a mixture of water, electrolytes, bile pigments (largely bilirubin), bile acids, cholesterol, phospholipids, albumin and immunoglobulins. This composition allows it to have a broad range of physiological functions including lipid digestion and absorption, immunological defence, excretion of endogenous compounds and removal of xenobiotics.

Formation of bilirubin

The body produces approximately 250–400 mg of bilirubin daily, primarily from the breakdown of haemoglobin:

- Haem is enzymatically degraded releasing iron, carbon monoxide and biliverdin (green), which is subsequently reduced to bilirubin (yellow) by the enzyme biliverdin reductase.

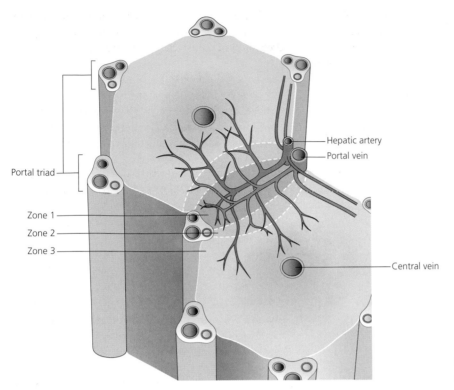

Hepatic artery
Portal vein

Portal triad

Zone 1
Zone 2
Zone 3

Central vein

Figure G Functional liver acinus.

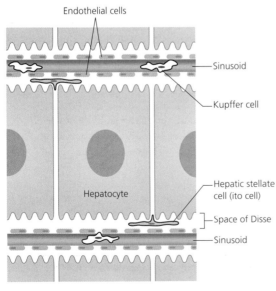

Endothelial cells

Sinusoid

Kupffer cell

Hepatocyte

Hepatic stellate cell (ito cell)

Space of Disse

Sinusoid

Figure H Anatomy of the hepatic sinusoid.

• This unconjugated bilirubin is water insoluble and therefore circulates in plasma tightly bound to albumin.

• Conjugation of bilirubin with glucoronic acid occurs in hepatocytes and confers water solubility, allowing efficient excretion in the bile (Fig. I).

• Following conjugation, the major bilirubin pigment is bilirubin diglucoronide; bilirubin monoglucoronide and unconjugated bilirubin account for less than 20% of the pigments.

• Conjugated bilirubin is transported from the hepatocyte to the biliary canaliculus by an adenosine triphosphate (ATP) dependent export pump.

A number of inherited conditions are caused by defects in the process of bilirubin conjugation and excretion from the liver (Table A).

Enterohepatic circulation

Conjugated bilirubin is water soluble and therefore there is little reabsorption in the small intestine. In the colon, bacterial glucoronidases hydrolyse conjugated bilirubin, forming urobilinogen, a non-polar substance that is reabsorbed in the intestine. This is re-excreted in the bile (major fraction) or urine (minor fraction). Although

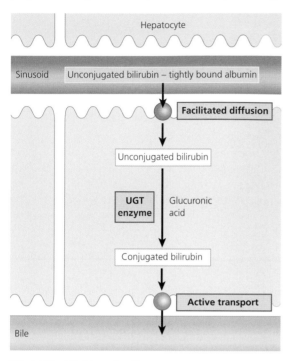

Figure I The bilirubin conjugation process.

urobilinogen is colourless, its oxidised product urobilin contributes to the colour of stool and urine (Fig. J). Urobilinogen is further converted to stercobilin in the colon.

Clinical implications of bilirubin metabolism (Table B)

• Prehepatic jaundice causes an increase in unconjugated bilirubin; this is bound to albumin and is not detected in the urine, which remains a normal colour. The stool colour is normal.

   ○ In haemolysis there is increased delivery of bilirubin to the gut resulting in increased production of urobilinogen.

   ○ In conjugating enzyme defects there is reduced formation of urobilinogen.

• In obstructive jaundice there is disruption to the enterohepatic circulation, urobilinogen and urobilin are absent from the urine, and stercobilin is absent from the stools, which become pale. The urine becomes dark because there is excess conjugated bilirubin in the blood which is water soluble and therefore passes through the renal glomerular filter into the urine (Fig. K).

• In hepatocellular damage, there is impairment of conjugation within the hepatocytes and transport of conjugated bilirubin from the hepatocytes to the bile duct resulting in raised plasma concentration of unconjugated and conjugated bilirubin. Urobilinogen re-excretion by

Table A Disorders of bilirubin formation.

Condition	Inheritance	Defect	Notes
Gilbert's syndrome	Autosomal recessive*	Decreased bilirubin glucoronidation Defects in the promoter of UDP glucoronyl transferase have been identified	Common, affects 5–10% of the population Clinically entirely benign condition
Crigler–Najjar syndrome	Autosomal recessive		Rare Unconjugated hyperbilirubinaemia
Type 1		Absence of UDP glucoronyl transferase	Severe hyperbilirubinaemia, death in neonatal period
Type 2		Reduction in UDP glucoronyl transferase	Moderate hyperbilirubinaemia
Dubin–Johnson syndrome	Autosomal recessive	Absent expression of ATP-dependent export pump	Uncommon Conjugated hyperbilirubinaemia
Rotor's syndrome	Autosomal recessive	Unknown	Rare Conjugated hyperbilirubinaemia

* Gilbert's syndrome is generally considered to be an autosomal recessive disorder; however, there are references in the literature suggesting autosomal dominant inheritance.
ATP, adenosine triphosphate; UDP, uridine diphosphate.

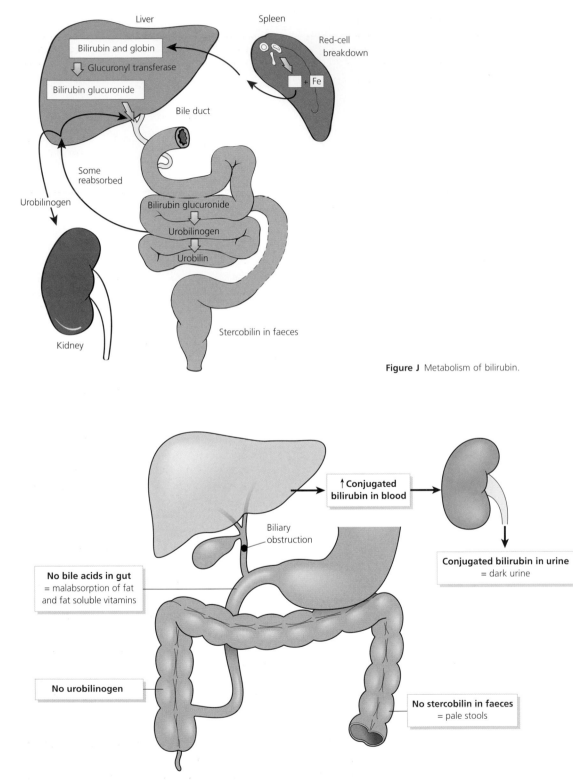

Figure J Metabolism of bilirubin.

Figure K Obstructive jaundice.

Table B Clinical findings in different types of jaundice.

	Prehepatic haemolysis	Prehepatic conjugation defects	Hepatic	Posthepatic
Serum bilirubin	Unconjugated	Unconjugated	Conjugated and unconjugated	Conjugated
Urine colour	Normal	Normal	May be dark	Dark
Urinalysis	Elevated urobilinogen	Urobilinogen low or absent	Elevated urobilinogen	No urobilinogen Bilirubin present
Stool colour	Normal	Normal	May be pale	Pale

the liver is also affected, resulting in increased excretion in the urine.

Bile acids

Bile acids are synthesised in the liver from cholesterol. They are conjugated in the liver with amino acids (glycine or taurine) to form bile salts, which are excreted in bile. In the intestine bile salts are reabsorbed in the terminal ileum. The small fraction that enters the colon is converted to secondary bile salts by the action of colonic bacteria, which then enters the enterohepatic circulation. There are a number of functions of bile acids/salts:

• Contribution to secretion of cholesterol and phospholipids from the liver.
• Major solute of bile and contributes to bile flow.
• Allows excretion of lipid-soluble substances by forming micelles.
• Absorption and digestion of lipids, including lipid-soluble vitamins.
• Signalling properties in the hepatocyte and biliary epithelium (e.g. regulate expression of genes responsible for bile synthesis and metabolism).

Clinical implications of bile acids

• In biliary obstruction a reduction in bile salt excretion may cause deficiencies in the absorption of fat-soluble vitamins (A, D, E and K). In the context of liver disease, this may result in prolonged coagulation because of the resulting low levels of vitamin K.
• Disease or resection of the terminal ileum interrupts the normal enterohepatic circulation of bile salts. The increased delivery of bile salts to the colon may cause diarrhoea and result in electrolyte and water loss in the faeces.

Gallbladder function

The principle functions of the gallbladder are the storage and concentration of bile. In response to neurological reflexes and the gut hormone cholecystokinin (CCK) it contracts to release bile in the duodenum. Although it is not essential for bile secretion, it concentrates bile by up to 10-fold and patients who have had their gallbladder removed may develop upper gastrointestinal symptoms such as oesophagitis or gastritis related to the continuous flow of bile into the gut.

Central metabolic functions of the liver

The liver is a central hub for the metabolism of carbohydrates, protein and lipids. Within the sinusoid there are zones where different metabolic processes are concentrated.

Glucose metabolism

The liver has a pivotal role in glucose homeostasis. Following a meal approximately 25% of the glucose content is metabolised in the liver – stored as glycogen, oxidised or converted to fat. The liver maintains plasma blood glucose levels by two distinct pathways, gluconeogensis (converts carbon-containing compounds such as amino acids into glucose) and glycogenolysis (conversion of glycogen into glucose).

• The homeostasis between glucose storage and glucose production is relative to the concentrations of the hormones insulin (produced in pancreatic β cells) and glucagon (produced in pancreatic alpha cells).
• A raised insulin:glucagon ratio inhibits gluconeogensis and promotes glycogen synthesis.
• A reduced insulin:glucagon ratio promotes gluconeogenesis and inhibits glycogen synthesis.

Protein and amino acid metabolism

The liver has diverse functions pertaining to protein metabolism, including:
- The synthesis and degradation of amino acids and proteins including albumin, globulin and fibrinogen.
- The production of ammonia from the deamination of amino acids and subsequent conversion to urea (via the intermediates ornithine, citruline and arginine) by the urea cycle, which occurs exclusively in the liver.
- The production of glucose from the main 'gluconeogenic' amino acids alanine and glutamine.
- The production of fatty acids from 'ketogenic' amino acids, e.g. leucine and lysine.
- The formation of glutathione (important antioxidant role) and creatine (an important energy source in skeletal muscle which spontaneously breaks down to creatinine), which is dependent upon amino acid metabolism within the liver.

Lipid metabolism

Cholesterol degradation and excretion is dependent on the liver. Due to their insolubility, the transport of cholesterol and triglycerides is reliant on lipoproteins (Fig. L).

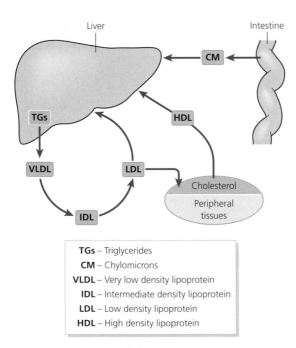

TGs – Triglycerides
CM – Chylomicrons
VLDL – Very low density lipoprotein
IDL – Intermediate density lipoprotein
LDL – Low density lipoprotein
HDL – High density lipoprotein

Figure L Lipid transport and the liver.

- Chylomicrons, very low density lipoproteins (VLDLs), low density lipoproteins (LDLs) and high density lipoproteins (HDLs) are all part of the apolipoprotein family.
- With increasing density, there is reducing size, reduced cholesterol content and increased protein content of the particles.
- Lipids are transported from the intestine to the liver in chylomicrons.
- The liver exports fatty acids as VLDLs, which releases free fatty acids by the action of peripheral lipoprotein lipases.
- LDLs are taken up by target tissues by endocytosis or by LDL-receptor-mediated uptake in the liver.
- HDLs transport cholesterol back to the liver for elimination (Fig. L).
- Cholesterol within the liver is excreted as bile salts (see above).

Clinical implications of disordered metabolism in liver disease

- Glycogen storage diseases are inherited disorders caused by deficiency of enzymes that catalyse the conversion of glycogen and glucose. In the hepatic forms this can result in hypoglycaemia, hepatomegaly (due to excess glycogen in the liver) and growth retardation.
- In severe acute liver failure, hypoglycaemia occurs because of the inability of the liver to maintain plasma glucose by either gluconeogenesis or glycogenolysis.
- In cirrhosis there may be a combination of reduced glycogen reserves (less glycogenolysis), which is compensated for by increased gluconeogenesis.
- Insulin resistance, altered carbohydrate and lipid metabolism (resulting in increased free fatty acid efflux into the liver) and inflammatory cytokines contribute to the condition of non-alcoholic fatty liver disease (NAFLD).
- Reduced muscle mass in chronic liver disease is a reflection of reduced nutritional intake but also increased catabolism (may reflect increased proteolysis for the provision of gluconeogenic amino acids).
- The inability of the liver to adequately metabolise ammonia (because of increased portosystemic shunting and reduced elimination in the urea cycle) may have an important aetiological role in the development of hepatic encephalopathy.

Drug metabolism

The liver plays a major role in drug metabolism and elimination. Drugs are taken up by the liver and then processed by a number of enzymatic reactions:

1 Phase 1 metabolism alters the structural integrity of the drug by enzymes, including the cytochrome P450 system. The resultant metabolite is not necessarily detoxified and may in fact be more active (e.g. the metabolite *N*-acetyl-*p*-benzoquionimine (NAPQI) produced by phase I metabolism of paracetamol is hepatotoxic). The efficacy of this system is determined by genetic factors and also induction by other drugs.

2 Phase 2 metabolism results in conjugation of the metabolite, which can detoxify and increase solubility for excretion.

Liver disease can affect drug metabolism in a number of ways. Firstly, portosystemic shunting will reduce metabolism of drugs within the liver and, secondly, reduced albumin synthesis will alter the ratio of unbound : bound drug in the plasma.

Immune function

The vascular supply through the liver and the arrival of potentially pathogenic substances, via the portal vein from the gut, makes the liver an important immunological site. The liver has diverse immune functions:

• Kupffer cells are resident macrophages located in the hepatic sinusoids. They have important roles in phagocytosis, cytokine and chemokine release and activation of other cells including the hepatic stellate cell.

• In addition to the trafficking of activated lymphocytes from the circulation into the liver there is also a specific intrahepatic population of lymphocytes, natural killer cells (part of the innate immune system) and dendritic cells (which present antigen to T cells).

• Immune tolerance may have particular relevance for the liver in view of the high antigenic load it receives from the gut. There is a balance of protecting against excessive immune activation (e.g. autoimmunity) versus allowing the persistence of pathogens (chronic viral hepatitis).

• Secretory IgA in the bile contributes to hepatobiliary and gastrointestinal mucosal immunity. Raised serum levels of IgA are found in alcoholic liver disease; the exact reason is uncertain but there is some evidence that alcohol can disrupt the gastrointestinal epithelial barrier resulting in greater antigen translocation across the gut.

Pathophysiological processes affecting the liver

Acute inflammation

The causes of acute hepatitis are broad (Box A). Damage may occur by hepatocellular necrosis or apoptosis (pro-

---

Box A Causes of acute inflammation

• Infection:
  ○ hepatitis A, B, C, D and E
  ○ Epstein–Barr virus, cytomegalovirus, herpes simplex virus
• Drugs: paracetamol, ecstasy, herbal remedies
• Vascular:
  ○ ischaemia
  ○ Budd–Chiari syndrome (obstruction of the large hepatic veins)
• Metabolic: Wilson's disease
• Malignancy: malignant infiltration of the liver
• Pregnancy: acute fatty liver of pregnancy
• Miscellaneous:
  ○ autoimmune hepatitis
  ○ sepsis
  ○ *Amanita* mushroom poisoning
  ○ heat stroke

---

grammed cell death). The liver injury can result in asymptomatic transaminitis (deranged liver function tests but no clinical signs or symptoms), anicteric hepatitis (no jaundice but symptoms such as fever, vomiting, right upper quadrant discomfort, etc.), icteric hepatitis (jaundice but no encephalopathy) or fulminant liver failure (coagulopathy and hepatic encephalopathy). The liver has a remarkable capacity for regeneration and the balance of this regeneration versus injury will determine the outcome:

• Acute hepatitis with complete resolution.
• Fulminant liver failure.
• Chronic liver injury leading to fibrosis.

Acute liver failure

The term acute liver failure implies the presence of encephalopathy in the context of an acute liver injury. The following classification is often used:

• Hyperacute liver failure: encephalopathy within 7 days of jaundice.
• Acute liver failure: encephalopathy between 8 and 28 days after the onset of jaundice.
• Subacute liver failure: encephalopathy between 5 and 12 weeks after the onset of jaundice.

Inadequate liver function results in reduced hepatic metabolism of ammonia and contributes to the development of encephalopathy. The resulting excessive ammonia is metabolised in the brain causing accumulation of glutamine in astrocytes, raised cellular osmotic pressure and cerebral oedema. Oedema is further accentuated by an increase in cerebral blood flow due to disruption of the normal autoregulatory mechanisms. If the intracranial pressure becomes elevated above a critical threshold cerebral perfusion may be compromised and brainstem herniation can occur.

In addition to encephalopathy other clinical manifestations include renal dysfunction, hyperdynamic circulation (increased cardiac output and reduced systemic vascular resistance), hyperventilation, prolonged coagulation, sepsis (including fungal infections) and hypoglycaemia.

Chronic liver injury, fibrosis and cirrhosis

Chronic liver injury can result from a spectrum of insults (Table C) and frequently leads to fibrosis, an innate wound healing response of the body. Fibrosis usually takes several years to develop but can occasionally develop rapidly over months (e.g childhood biliary atresia, certain drug-induced liver diseases and the post liver transplantation setting). Liver fibrosis is characterised by the deposition of extracellular matrix (scar tissue) consisting of collagens, hyaluronic acid, proteoglycans and matrix glycoproteins. The hepatic stellate cell, residing in the space of Disse within the sinusoids, plays a central role in secreting collagen scar tissue. Progressive injury eventually leads to the formation of fibrous tissue bands separating nodules of regenerative hepatocytes, when it is known as cirrhosis. Cirrhosis may be defined as micronodular (small nodules less than 3 mm) or macronodular (Fig. M).

The development of cirrhosis alters haemodynamics within and outside the liver. Extracellular matrix deposition within the sinusoids causes a loss of the normal fenestration (analogous to changing from a porous pipe

Table C Examples of chronic liver injury.

Category	Aetiology	Notes
Infection	Hepatitis B (HBV) Hepatitis C (HCV) Schistosomiasis	HBV is the commonest cause of chronic liver disease worldwide
Metabolic	Non-alcoholic steatohepatitis (NASH) Haemochromatosis Wilson's disease Alpha-1 antitrypsin deficiency Glycogen storage disease Tyrosinaemia Porphyria	NASH is becoming a leading cause of liver disease due to the increasing prevalence of obesity and insulin resistance
Vascular	Veno-occlusive disease Budd–Chiari syndrome Cardiac failure	Budd–Chiari syndrome is a result of obstruction to the hepatic venous outflow, often as a result of a thrombosis; classically patients present with hepatic engorgement and ascites
Immunological	Autoimmune hepatitis Primary biliary cirrhosis	Long-term immunosuppression is often required in autoimmune hepatitis as recurrent inflammatory flares may be asymptomatic and lead to cirrhosis
Biliary disease	Primary sclerosing cholangitis Biliary obstruction (intra- or extrahepatic)	Longstanding biliary obstruction can result in secondary biliary cirrhosis
Drugs and toxins	Alcohol Methotrexate Amiodarone	
Miscellaneous	Malnutrition Ischaemia Sarcoidosis	Hepatic sarcoidosis is an example of a granulomatous liver disease. The granulomas, when present, are non-caseating (cf. tuberculosis)

Nodules > 3 mm

Nodules < 3 mm

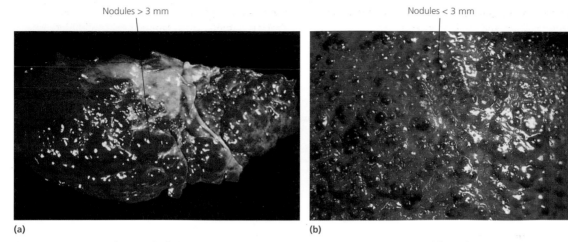

(a)

(b)

Figure M Macroscopic photograph of a liver showing cirrhosis. (a) Macronodular cirrhosis. (b) Micronodular cirrhosis.

to a lead pipe) and subsequent reduced filtration and hypoxia. Furthermore, the release of angiogenic factors stimulates new blood vessel formation (neoangiogenesis) within the fibrous tissue. The resulting intrahepatic shunting of blood contributes to the reduction in hepatic function that occurs in advanced fibrosis and cirrhosis. The vascular resistance in the liver increases due to a combination of structural alterations (e.g. scar tissue and nodules) and dynamic alterations (e.g. contraction of the hepatic stellate cell) in the liver parenchyma. The rise in intrahepatic vascular resistance contributes to the elevation in portal venous pressure that frequently complicates cirrhosis.

Regeneration

The human liver is the only organ able to regenerate lost tissue. A whole liver can regenerate from as little as 25% of its normal size. The mechanisms are not entirely clear but probably involve hepatocytes entering cell cycle in response to signals including growth factors and cytokines. There is also evidence for bipotential stem cells (oval cells) that can differentiate into either hepatocytes or cholangiocytes. Once a liver has become chronically damaged and has developed extensive fibrosis its ability to regenerate becomes impaired, an important fact in selecting patients for surgical resection.

Neoplasia

Neoplasia is the abnormal proliferation of cells. It results when a cell becomes genetically altered so that it evades the normal controls on growth and proliferation. A neoplasm may be benign (e.g. adenoma) or malignant, when it is frequently called a cancer. Malignant neoplasms may invade and destroy surrounding tissues, they can spread (metastasise) and may kill the host. The liver is a frequent site of spread from other neoplasms, particularly those of the gastrointestinal tract and pancreas, which are drained by the portal venous system. Hepatic metastases may be solitary or multiple. Neoplasms relevant to the hepatobiliary system are demonstrated in Fig. N.

Multiple mechanisms are responsible for the genetic changes that occur in neoplasia. Eighty per cent of hepatocellular carcinomas (HCCs) occur on a background of cirrhosis, probably because the repeated cycles of inflammation, oxidative damage and repair result in genetic damage that predisposes to malignant change. Hepatitis B virus causes HCC by inducing cirrhosis but can also cause HCC in non-cirrhotic livers, which may be secondary to its ability to integrate into host cellular DNA. Risk factors for developing the commonest malignant neoplasms, HCC and cholangiocarcinoma, are shown in Box B.

The site of the neoplasm determines the characteristic of the disease presentation. For example, lesions in the biliary system frequently cause obstruction and present with jaundice, whereas lesions in the liver parenchyma rarely cause jaundice until late stages and are only picked up when disease is advanced unless they are detected incidentally or as a result of screening. Consequently, the prognosis of hepatobiliary malignant neoplasms is frequently poor.

Infection

Infection occurs when a microorganism enters a host and replicates there. Disease results when the microorganism

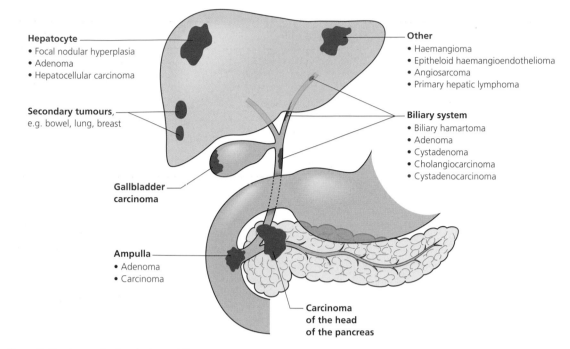

Figure N Neoplasms affecting the hepatobiliary system.

> **Box B Main aetiological factors for hepatobiliary carcinomas**
>
> **Hepatocellular carcinoma**
> - Cirrhosis (all causes but especially HBV, HCV, alcohol and haemochromatosis)
> - Hepatitis B virus (even in the absence of cirrhosis)
> - Aflatoxins from *Aspergillus flavus* and *A. parasiticus*
>
> **Cholangiocarcinoma**
> - Primary sclerosing cholangitis
> - Chronic gallstones
> - Liver fluke (*Clonorchis sinensis*)

causes damage to the host during the process of infection. The liver is frequently involved in infection, either as the primary target organ or as part of a generalised multiorgan process. The portal venous circulation and the biliary tract provide potential routes for infectious agents to access the liver from the gastrointestinal tract. In addition, the rich vascular supply to the liver results in it being susceptible to infection as a consequence of systemic infections. Many different classes of microorganism can result in hepatic infection (Table D).

Clinical impact of infection

The clinical impact of hepatic infection is determined by a number of factors including the site of infection, the mechanism by which the organism causes damage and the extent of the host's response to the invading organism.

Site of infection

The clinical features of hepatic infection are determined by the site of infection.

Liver parenchyma

- *Hepatitis*: Hepatitis is the term given for inflammation of the liver parenchyma; infection, in particular viral infection, is an important cause. Viruses may cause hepatitis as a primary manifestation of infection (e.g. hepatitis A to E) or as part of a more generalised systemic infection (e.g. cytomegalovirus, Ebstein–Barr virus, herpes simplex virus). Infectious hepatitis results in a spectrum of clinical syndromes ranging from subclinical infection, to clinical infection with or without jaundice, to acute liver failure with possible death (rare).
- *Abscess*: Abscesses in the liver are most frequently caused by bacteria, although amoebic abscesses may be seen in travellers to endemic areas and fungal abscesses

Table D Agents causing infection of the liver.

Virus	Bacteria	Protozoa	Parasite	Fungus
Hepatitis A to E	Gram-negative bacteria, e.g. *Escherichia coli*	*Entamoeba histolytica*	*Echinococcus* (hydatid disease) Schistosomiasis	*Candida* *
Cytomegalovirus		*Pneumocystis carinii* *		*Cryptococcus* *
Ebstein–Barr virus	*Klebsiella, Pseudomonas,* enterococci, etc.		*Ascaris lumbricoides*	
Herpes simplex virus	*Mycobacteria* species		Flukes, e.g. *Clonorchis sinensis*	
Yellow fever virus	Leptospirosis			

* Usually only seen as disseminated infection in an immunocompromised host.

can occur in the immunocompromised. Typical symptoms are malaise, anorexia, fever and right upper quadrant discomfort.

• *Tuberculosis*: Liver involvement in tuberculosis (TB) is common, histological abnormalities being seen in up to 75% of patients with pulmonary TB as a consequence of haematogenous spread from the primary source. Diffuse parenchymal hepatic TB is the most common form, characterised by small (<1 mm) granulomas throughout the liver parenchyma. Less commonly, focal hepatic TB occurs with a tuberculous liver abscess or tuberculoma. These lesions are usually larger (>2 mm) and may be solitary or multiple.

Biliary system

• *Cholangitis*: Cholangitis is the result of infection within the biliary system. It frequently occurs when there is obstruction to biliary drainage, for example by impaction of a gallstone in the bile duct, with ascending infection behind the obstruction. Cholangitis may also occur as a complication of surgery or endoscopic instrumentation of the biliary tract (e.g. endoscopic retrograde cholangiopancreatography (ERCP)). The invading microorganisms arise from the gastrointestinal tract (e.g. *Escherichia coli*). Spread of the microorganisms into the liver parenchyma may occur with development of hepatic abscesses. Patients with ascending cholangitis typically present with fever, jaundice and right upper quadrant pain (Charcot's triad*).

• *Gallbladder empyema*: Bacterial contamination of the gallbladder may result in production of a purulent inflammatory exudate resulting in a gallbladder

empyema. This usually results from obstruction of the cystic duct, typically by gallstones. The patient is unwell and requires antibiotics and urgent drainage or removal of the gallbladder.

• *Parasitic infection*: Some parasites can infect the biliary system in humans. *Fasciola hepatica* is a sheep fluke found in parts of Europe including England. Flukes hatch in the small intestine, penetrate the intestinal wall, cross the peritoneal cavity and enter the hepatic parenchyma, eventually reaching the biliary tree. Here mature worms produce eggs in the bile duct, which enter the small intestine and are passed from the body in faeces. Infection may be asymptomatic or may mimic ascending cholangitis. Tapeworms of the *Echinococcus* genus can infect the liver. Humans become infected by ingesting eggs that hatch in the intestine and migrate to the liver and other organs. Large complex cysts (hydatid cysts) can form in the liver which may be asymptomatic or cause symptoms related to pressure. *Clonorchis sinensis* is a liver fluke most commonly seen in Asia. The adult flukes live in the bile ducts and release eggs that can result in severe inflammation and fibrosis. Infestation with this parasite has been linked to the development of cholangiocarcinoma.

Blood vessels

Schistosomiasis (bilharzia). *Schistosoma mansoni* and *S. japonica* cause liver disease. Cercariae from infected water enter humans by penetrating unbroken skin. They migrate through the venous system to the liver and mesenteric veins where the adult worms mature and produce eggs. Eggs retained in the mesenteric vessels produce intense inflammation and fibrosis. Hepatic schistosomiasis results in fibrosis around the portal veins and a granulomatous inflammation within the hepatic parenchyma. Patients are not cirrhotic but the severe periportal

---

*Jean-Martin Charcot (1825–1893), French neurologist.

fibrosis leads to portal hypertension and subsequent development of splenomegaly, ascites and varices.

Mechanisms of disease

Disease may result from direct damage caused by the invading microorganism itself or indirectly via the host's response to the microorganism, or a combination of the two.

Direct damage

Only a few organisms cause hepatic disease by directly damaging the host. Some of the viruses that cause haemorrhagic fevers (e.g. yellow fever or Rift Valley fever) can cause direct hepatocyte necrosis. As a part of a multisystem illness these viruses diffusely infect hepatocytes which are destroyed by the replicating virus, resulting in death in up to 50% of cases. Hepatitis viruses may in some circumstances cause disease by a direct cytopathic effect but the main mechanism of disease is by indirect damage (see below).

Indirect damage

• *Inflammation*: The presence of microorganisms in tissues frequently elicits an inflammatory reaction as part of the host response to attempt to destroy and eradicate the invading organism. Often this inflammation itself leads to damage that produces disease. An example of this is the inflammatory response to schistosomal eggs mentioned above. The presence of the eggs in the portal vessels induces a granulomatous inflammatory reaction which eventually results in healing by fibrosis. Disease is then caused by the fibrotic narrowing of the portal vessels, resulting in portal hypertension.

• *Immune response*: Hepatitis viruses classically cause disease by inducing an immune response. The extent and severity of the disease is related to the strength of the immune response to the virus and varies considerably between individuals. This is best illustrated by hepatitis B virus (HBV) infection. Infection acquired as a neonate, when the immune system is immature, almost invariably results in chronic carriage of the virus. Individuals have high levels of viraemia but remain well with normal liver blood tests and normal liver histology. Individuals who acquire HBV infection as an adult, however, may have a more developed immunological response and develop symptomatic hepatitis. Liver blood tests may be abnormal and biopsy reveals hepatocyte necrosis with lymphocyte infiltration of the liver parenchyma. In the most extreme example of symptomatic hepatitis B infection, the immune response is so intense that total hepatocyte necrosis occurs and the liver fails; fortunately this is very rare.

Immunosuppression

Despite the fact that the immune system is responsible for a large component of the injury caused by viruses such as hepatitis B and C, these viruses actually cause more damage if the patient is immunosuppressed, for example in human immunodeficiency virus (HIV) infection and following liver transplantation. In this situation it seems that the virus is capable of directly damaging hepatocytes, illustrating the fact that it is the complex interplay between both the virus and the host response to it that dictates the pathology caused.

Immunosuppression also increases the likelihood of opportunistic infections. Fungal infections such as with *Candida* are rarely seen in those with an intact immune system but may occur in patients who are immunosuppressed. Other infections such as mycobacterial infections (*Mycobacterium tuberculosis*, *M. avium-intracellulare*, *M. kansaii*) and *Pneumocystis carinii* infection of the liver may be seen in those with a severely compromised immune system.

The liver and systemic infection
Infection in liver failure

The liver is a key component of the host immune response to infection. It produces many of the proteins involved in the innate response against infection, e.g. proteins of the complement cascade. In addition it contains a resident macrophage population, the Kupffer cells, which play a significant role in the removal of toxins and foreign substances from the portal blood. Severe hepatic injury, either in acute liver failure or in cirrhosis, results in impairment of these hepatic defences. This leads to an increased susceptibility of the host to infections, particularly bacterial and fungal infections. Infection can occur anywhere but is frequently cultured from blood, urine and sputum. A common and clinically important example is spontaneous infection of ascites from bacteria translocating across the gastrointestinal lumen (spontaneous bacterial peritonitis).

Sepsis-related change in liver function

Infection in extrahepatic sites can produce changes in liver function. Hepatic dysfunction has many causes including hypoxia and decreased hepatic perfusion seen in systemic sepsis and release of cytokines and free radicals by activated Kupffer cells.

Drug toxicity

Many drugs in common use can cause toxic effects on the liver ranging from mild subclinical reactions to fulminant hepatic failure. Patients frequently take multiple drugs which can make it difficult to identify the hepatotoxic agent. A careful history including dose, route of administration, duration of use and concomitant medication must be taken. As well as enquiring about prescribed medications (current and in the past 3 months), it is also important to consider herbal and over the counter medications which are frequently implicated in drug-induced liver disease. Risk factors for drug-induced liver injury are given in Box C.

Mechanisms of hepatotoxicity

• Some drugs produce liver injury in a predictable, dose-dependent manner in most individuals (e.g. paracetamol excess). The injury characteristically affects one area of the liver lobule, for example paracetamol causes zone 3 or centrilobular necrosis. The damage is frequently not caused by the drug itself but by a toxic effect of a reactive metabolite causing oxidative damage to cellular proteins and nucleic acids and disrupting their function.

• Other drugs result in unpredictable or idiosyncratic liver injury that is not dose dependent (e.g. isoniazid). The liver injury is more diffuse, affecting the whole liver lobule. Immunological mechanisms may be involved including a hypersensitivity reaction that develops after 1–4 weeks and is characterised by fever, rash, eosinophilia and lymphocytosis. This may be a result of alterations in endogenous proteins, by binding of the drug or its metabolites, which then provoke an autoimmune response. Some may develop autoantibodies. Withdrawing the drug may terminate this response but in some cases a chronic autoimmune hepatitis may develop. The reaction recurs quickly if the drug is readministered.

Patterns of drug-induced hepatotoxicity

There are many patterns of drug-induced injury (Table E). Two main categories are commonly found:

• *Hepatocellular damage*: Damage to the hepatocyte may be acute or chronic. The types of injury vary including necrosis, steatosis and non-specific hepatitis, which

---

Box C Risk factors for hepatic drug injury

• *Liver disease*: drug metabolism is impaired due to:
  ○ reduction in hepatic blood flow with decreased first-pass metabolism
  ○ impaired oxidative metabolism and glucuronidation
  ○ reduced albumin synthesis altering the ratio of unbound:bound drug in the plasma
• *Age*: older age increases the risk of hepatotoxicity due to:
  ○ reduced liver blood flow
  ○ decreased activity of the cytochrome P450 system
  ○ reduced renal clearance
• *Sex*: some drug reactions are more common in females (e.g. nitrofurantoin and non-steroidal anti-inflammatory drugs)
• *Nutrition*:
  ○ obesity may predispose to hepatotoxicity through prolonged exposure to fat-soluble drugs
  ○ malnutrition may impair glutathione synthesis, increasing the risk of paracetamol (acetaminophen) toxicity
• *Other drugs*: enzyme induction by drugs such as anticonvulsants, isoniazid and ethanol increase the risk of drug-related hepatotoxicity

---

Table E Patterns of drug-related liver injury.

Mechanism	Drug examples
Hepatocellular injury	
Necrosis	Paracetamol
Steatosis	Sodium valproate, ethanol
Hepatitis	Isoniazid, methyl dopa
Granulomas	Isoniazid, carbamazepine
Cholestatic injury	
Acute	Co-amoxiclav, oestrogens
Chronic	Chlorpromazine, phenytoin
Vascular	
Hepatic vein occlusion	Oestrogens
Veno-occlusive disease	Cytotoxic agents
Peliosis hepatis	Anabolic steroids
Nodular regenerative hyperplasia	Azathioprine
Fibrosis	Methotrexate
Neoplasms	
Adenoma	Oestrogens
Hepatocellular carcinoma	Oestrogens, vinyl chloride
Angiosarcoma	Vinyl chloride

may resemble autoimmune hepatitis or a granulomatous hepatitis.

• *Cholestatic damage*: Intrahepatic cholestasis is a common manifestation of drug-induced liver injury. Symptoms may mimic extrahepatic biliary obstruction but there is an absence of duct dilatation on ultrasound imaging. Histology may reveal evidence of inflammation in the portal regions which can be accompanied by destruction and loss of bile ducts.

Clinical features of drug-induced liver injury and management

Symptoms are generally non-specific, making diagnosis difficult and a high index of suspicion required to diagnose drug-induced liver injury. Many drugs cause an illness similar to viral hepatitis with a prodrome of nausea and anorexia followed by abdominal pain and jaundice. Drugs that cause hypersensitivity reactions may cause fever, rash and arthralgia.

Diagnosis may be difficult since the clinical symptoms and any changes in laboratory indices are non-specific. Often the diagnosis is suspected merely because the patient improves when the drug is discontinued; however, some drug-related injuries continue to deteriorate despite drug withdrawal. Furthermore, patients are often on multiple drugs and have serious underlying illnesses making it difficult to identify the cause of liver injury. The key component to making a diagnosis is a careful and thorough history of recent and past drug exposure including non-prescribed medications.

The main treatment is withdrawal of the injurious agent and supportive care for symptoms such as pruritus. Most patients will recover completely although a few continue to deteriorate, and in some liver transplantation may ultimately be necessary.

Vascular pathophysiology in liver disease
Hepatic ischaemia

The liver has a dual blood supply with approximately 70–80% of blood flow derived from the portal vein and the remainder from the hepatic artery. Therefore the liver is relatively well protected from ischaemia due to systemic hypotension. However, the combination of hepatic congestion and hypotension can provoke hepatic ischaemia. The most common scenario for this to occur is in cardiac patients, where longstanding cardiac failure causes hepatic congestion, and who then have an acute hypotensive episode; in essence there is 'forward failure' and 'backward congestion'. Hypoxia or anaemia will further aggravate hepatic ischaemia.

• Acute hepatic ischaemia may be asymptomatic and associated with a large increase in transaminases (can approach 1000 iU/L) and reduced synthetic function. In the majority of cases this will resolve with conservative treatment within 7 days but in a small proportion of cases acute liver failure may ensue.

• In chronic cardiac congestion liver cirrhosis may result. The resulting congestion in the centilobular region and sinusoidal dilatation leads to the 'nutmeg' appearance seen at autopsy.

Portal hypertension and haemodynamics in cirrhosis

Portal hypertension is defined by an elevated portal pressure greater than the normal value of 1–5 mmHg. In general, portal pressure becomes clinically significant above a level of 12 mmHg. The major complications of portal hypertension include ascites, gastrointestinal haemorrhage and renal dysfunction. Of these, gastroin-

---

Box D The haemodynamics of liver cirrhosis

• Reduced blood pressure and increased heart rate:
  ○ low blood pressure due to reduced resistance of the peripheral circulation (systemic vascular resistance)
  ○ cardiac output and pulse rate may rise in early cirrhosis due to activation of the sympathetic nervous system
• Increased total blood volume but reduced central blood volume:
  ○ increased renal water and sodium retention
  ○ increased ADH release
  ○ splanchnic arterial vasodilatation results in pooling of blood in the splanchnic circulation
• Reduced renal blood flow:
  ○ risk of hepatorenal syndrome
• Hepatic venous pressure gradient:
  ○ the pressure across the sinusoids is known as the hepatic venous pressure gradient and is the pressure difference between the hepatic vein and portal vein. In cirrhosis, there is a relationship between this gradient and the development of complications, e.g. bleeding from varices
  ○ changes in liver architecture increase the resistance of blood flow within the liver
  ○ increased blood flow in the portal vein (due to pooling of blood in splanchnic circulation) will also increase portal hypertension
(Pressure = Resistance × Flow)

testinal haemorrhage is the most dramatic and occurs frequently. Prospective studies suggest that 90% of patients with cirrhosis will develop oesophageal varices and a third of these will bleed. Ascites can occur insidiously and it is associated with a 2-year survival of 50%; therefore it represents a landmark event in the evolution of cirrhosis. The normal haemodynamics are altered in cirrhosis, as outlined in Box D, and this underpins many of the complications of portal hypertension. Overall there is increased sodium and water, but the fluid is in the 'wrong compartment' and the homeostatic mechanisms the body employs to correct this, e.g activation of the rennin–angiotensin system, exacerbates the vicious cycle of events.

Approach to the patient

History

Except for patients who are extremely ill, the taking of a thorough and careful medical history should precede examination and treatment. An accurate history will often suggest the correct diagnosis and determine what investigations are necessary. It is important to remember that the individual consulting a doctor may be nervous and apprehensive, so it is essential they are put at ease by a friendly greeting and made to feel the centre of the interviewer's interest.

Begin the interview by introducing yourself, giving your name and position and asking consent to take a history. Ask open questions and allow patients adequate opportunity to answer in their own words as this is more likely to direct you to the patient's underlying concerns rather than what you perceive their problem to be. Once you have allowed the patient to give their own account of their problems it may be necessary to ask a series of direct questions to clarify the patient's account and to extract further information regarding their previous health, family history and social matters.

Presenting complaint

The history begins with asking about the patient's main complaint. Begin with an open question such as 'What is the main problem with your health?' or 'When were you last completely well?' Patients may have more than one presenting complaint. Record each presenting symptom in their own words rather than using medical interpretations of what was said. It is important to be sure you know what the patient means since their interpretation of medical terms may be different to yours. For instance, a patient reporting a stomach ache may not be referring to a problem in the upper gastrointestinal tract and could be describing a sensation anywhere in the abdomen from the suprapubic region to epigastrium. Common hepatology presentations are given in Box E.

History of presenting symptom

After eliciting a patient's presenting complaint or complaints you should take a careful history of each one, establishing:
- The mode and time of onset.
- Progression of the symptom.
- Associated symptoms.
- The effect the symptom has on the patient's life.

In order to obtain this information it is necessary to combine a series of open and directed questions. Success in achieving this requires a lot of practice that can only be obtained by spending time talking to patients.

Jaundice

Jaundice refers to the yellow discolouration of the sclera or skin. It is caused by the presence of excess bilirubin in the blood, which is deposited in tissues of the body, particularly those that contain elastin. It is usually seen first in the sclerae, which are rich in elastic fibres, and in patients with dark skin this may be the only site that it can be recognised. Often the relatives or a doctor notices jaundice before the patient does. Jaundice can be classified into prehepatic, hepatic and posthepatic causes (Table F).

If a patient presents with jaundice the following questions should be asked:
- What is the colour of the urine and stools? (Pale stools and dark urine occur with intra- or extrahepatic biliary obstruction.)
- Is there a history of abdominal pain? (Gallstones, for example, can cause right upper quadrant pain and jaundice.)
- Is there a history of fever, sweats or rigors? (Suggests that the infection is either in the liver or biliary tree.)
- Does the patient itch? (Suggests obstruction to the bile flow.)

> **Box E Common presentations in hepatology**
>
> - Jaundice
> - Abdominal pain
> - Abdominal swelling
> - Gastrointestinal bleeding
> - Encephalopathy
> - Pruritus (itch)
> - Asymptomatic but referred due to the incidental finding of abnormal blood tests or imaging or picked up via screening for a relevant risk factor

Table F Classification and common causes of jaundice.

Prehepatic	Hepatic	Posthepatic
Haemolysis (increased bilirubin load for the liver cells)	Hepatitis (alcohol, viruses, drugs, immune-related damage, etc.)	Common bile duct stones
Conjugation abnormalities (congenital or acquired defects in conjugation)	Cirrhosis	Carcinoma (head of pancreas, bile duct, ampulla)
Large haematomas (increased bilirubin load)	Intrahepatic cholestasis (drugs, viruses, autoimmune)	Benign biliary stricture
		Pancreatitis

- Was there a prodromal illness? (May suggest viral hepatitis.)
- Is there a history of weight loss? (In an older patient this may suggest malignancy.)
- Has there been a recent outbreak? (Suggests viral hepatitis, e.g. infection with hepatitis A virus.)
- Is there a risk factor for viral hepatitis? For example, recent travel to an endemic country (e.g. in Africa or Asia), sexual exposure, recreational drug use or receipt of blood products.
- Has the patient taken any drugs?
- What is their alcohol consumption?
- Is there a family history of jaundice?

Abdominal pain

Abdominal pain is a common presentation with many causes. Careful history taking will steer investigation to the appropriate organ system and will often lead to the correct diagnosis. The following questions should be considered:

- *Site and radiation*: Ask the patient to point to the area affected by the pain and enquire about radiation of the pain. Liver and biliary pain usually affects the epigastrium and right upper quadrant of the abdomen. Hepatobiliary pain may radiate to the right shoulder tip due to diaphragmatic irritation. Sometimes the pain is only felt in the shoulder tip which can lead to difficulties in diagnosis as patients may be thought to have chest or rheumatological causes for the pain. Pancreatic pain is felt in the epigastrium and often radiates to the back.
- *Frequency and duration*: It is important to determine whether the pain is acute or chronic, when it began, how long it lasts and how often it occurs.
- *Character and pattern*: Pain that comes and goes in waves is related to peristaltic movements and is known as colic. It typically suggests pain related to the bowel and ureters. Whilst biliary pain is frequently called 'biliary colic' this is often a misnomer as biliary pain is in fact rarely colicky. Cystic duct obstruction tends to cause a severe pain in the epigastric region that is constant and can last for several hours. If cholecystitis develops, the inflammation causes the pain to shift to the right upper quadrant and to become more severe.
- *Exacerbating and relieving factors*: Biliary pain may be precipitated by consumption of fatty meals since the presence of fat in the gastrointestinal tract stimulates gallbladder contraction via production of the hormone cholecystokinin. Patients with pancreatic pain may obtain some relief by sitting up and leaning forward.
- *Associated symptoms*: Nausea and vomiting are common associated symptoms of biliary and pancreatic pain. Itch suggests obstruction to biliary flow which may reflect an intrahepatic or extrahepatic process.

Abdominal swelling

Persistent swelling of the abdomen often suggests fluid accumulation within the peritoneal cavity (ascites). Other causes of abdominal swelling must be considered (for instance fat, pregnancy, flatus, faeces, organomegaly and an abdominal tumour), but these can usually be differentiated from ascites from the history and subsequent physical examination.

If a patient is thought to have ascites, questions should be asked to try to differentiate other processes from a hepatic cause. For example, a diagnosis of heart failure might be suggested by symptoms of breathlessness, chest pain or a past history of ischaemic or valvular heart disease. A history of renal disease could suggest nephrotic syndrome and gynaecological or gastrointestinal symptoms may point to a malignant cause.

Gastrointestinal bleeding

Patients with liver disease may develop portal hypertension, which can lead to the development of anastomoses between the portal and systemic venous systems and the development of tortuous veins called varices. Haemorrhage may occur from these vessels and can be torrential and life threatening. Haematemesis (vomiting blood) indicates that the site of the bleeding is proximal to or at the duodenum. Whilst haematemesis in a patient with liver disease may be caused by bleeding from oesophago-gastric varices the other common causes of acute gastrointestinal bleeding should always be considered (Box F). Melaena refers to the passage of black, tarry stools and usually results from bleeding from the upper digestive tract, although right-sided colonic or small bowel lesions can occasionally be responsible. Haematochezia is the passage of bright red blood per rectum. It usually indicates a colonic cause such as diverticular disease, angiodysplasia or carcinoma. Patients with liver disease may develop rectal bleeding secondary to rectal varices and rarely patients can present with haematochezia caused by massive haemorrhage from the upper gastrointestinal tract in the absence of haematemesis.

Encephalopathy

Patients with liver disease may develop portosystemic encephalopathy, a neuropsychiatric syndrome with disturbance of cognition and conscious level. This condition occurs in both cirrhosis and acute liver failure. The mechanism is not fully understood but impaired metabolic function of the liver in combination with blood bypassing the liver through portosystemic collaterals, allows 'toxic' metabolites direct access to the brain to produce the encephalopathy. Patients will rarely recognise the presence of encephalopathy so friends and relatives should be interviewed and asked about alteration in personality, mood and concentration. An early symptom is reversal of the normal sleep pattern with daytime somnolence but an inability to sleep at night.

Pruritus

Patients with liver disease, particularly cholestasis, may describe intense itch which can be disabling. This is often worse in the peripheries and at night.

Past medical history

A thorough review of past medical and surgical history is a mandatory part of the history. Many medical and surgical conditions can predispose to liver and pancreatico-biliary disease. Examples include:
• A history of inflammatory bowel disease (either ulcerative colitis or Crohn's disease) could suggest a diagnosis of autoimmune hepatitis or primary sclerosing cholangitis.
• Surgical procedures could result in jaundice from the anaesthesia (e.g. halothane), from hypoxic damage to hepatocytes (secondary to hypotension) or from direct damage to the bile duct during abdominal surgery.
• A history of autoimmune diseases such as thyroid disease, rheumatoid arthritis or coeliac disease could indicate autoimmune liver disease.
• A history of diabetes, hypercholesterolaemia or obesity might suggest non-alcoholic fatty liver disease.
• A current or previous history of gallstones could indicate that abdominal pain is caused by gallstone pancreatitis or cholecystitis, or that jaundice is caused by stone migration into the common bile duct resulting in biliary obstruction.
• A history of diabetes, arthritis or cardiac dysrhythmia or cardiomyopathy could indicate haemochromatosis.

Box F Causes of haematemesis and melaena

Common causes
• Peptic ulcer disease (duodenal ulcer, gastric ulcer, erosions)
• Inflammation (oesophagitis, gastritis, duodenitis)
• Oesophageal and/or gastric varices
• Mallory–Weiss tear

Less common causes
• Dieulafoy lesion (ecstatic submucosal artery)
• Vascular abnormalities (angiodysplasia, arteriovenous malformations, gastric antral vascular ectasia)
• Aortoenteric fistula
• Gastric carcinoma or other neoplasm
• Bleeding diathesis
• Alternative origin, e.g. nasopharyngeal bleeding or haemoptysis

Medication history

A full enquiry into past and present medication is a mandatory part of any medical history. A large number of drugs can interfere with bilirubin metabolism or affect the liver directly, for example:
- Acute hepatitis can result from halothane, non-steroidal anti-inflammatory drugs or phenytoin.
- Cholestasis may occur from a sensitivity reaction to many antibiotics and antipsychotic medications.
- Overdose of paracetamol (acetaminophen) can lead to acute hepatocyte necrosis.
- Fatty liver can result from the use of tetracycline, steroids or sodium valproate.

As well as asking about prescription medications it is also important to specifically enquire about exposure to drugs obtained from other sources. Jaundice, hepatitis, cholestasis and even liver failure have been associated with the use of illicit drugs (e.g. ecstasy), over the counter agents, herbal remedies and substances obtained over the internet (e.g. anabolic steroids).

> **KEY POINT**
>
> - Non-prescription drugs are a frequent cause of liver disease or jaundice and should be specifically enquired about in anyone presenting with suspected liver pathology

Family history

A number of liver-related conditions can have a familial predisposition:
- A family history of jaundice may suggest haemolysis or familial hyperbilirubinaemia.
- If family members are affected by anaemia or have undergone a splenectomy, jaundice could be caused by an inheritied haemolytic anaemia.
- A relative with hepatitis B infection should alert you to the possibility of the patient being a chronic carrier of

that virus or a jaundiced patient having recently acquired that virus.
- A family member with a history of iron overload requiring venesection, diabetes, heart or joint disease should prompt consideration of a diagnosis of haemochromatosis.

Social history

The social history is particularly important when enquiring about potential liver disease since alcohol and viral hepatitis are common causes. A detailed alcohol history is mandatory and should ascertain the volume and type of alcohol a patient is drinking to try to calculate the amount of alcohol per week in units. Detailed enquiry is necessary since patients often try to conceal the actual amount from health care professionals. Furthermore, patients often genuinely underestimate their alcohol consumption as the percentage and volume of alcohol served has increased dramatically over the past two decades. For example, 20 years ago a typical glass of wine was 125 ml of 8% alcohol and contained 1 unit. Today a glass is more likely to be 175 ml or even 250 ml of 13–15% alcohol. Similarly beer used to be served as 3% alcohol but today is more likely to be 5% or even 9%. This needs to be borne in mind when estimating alcohol usage in units (Table G). Safe recommendations for weekly alcohol intake are less than 14 units for women and less than 21 units for men.

A full sexual history should be obtained, asking specifically about unprotected sex. As hepatitis B has an incubation period of up to 6 months and can produce chronic disease over many years it is important to enquire about risk factors that may have occurred a long time ago. A history of injections (e.g. intravenous drug use or tattooing) is important as hepatitis B and C can be transmitted in this way. It is not just sharing needles that can put people at risk of acquiring blood-borne viruses; sharing equipment used to prepare the drugs as well as using the intranasal route of drug administration are recognised risk factors for virus transmission. A

Table G Calculation of alcohol units.

	Wine				Beer		
	8%	12%	15%		3%	5%	9%
125 ml	1 unit	1.5 units	1.8 units	330 ml bottle	1 unit	1.7 units	3 units
175 ml	1.4 units	2.1 units	2.7 units	Pint (568 ml)	1.3 units	2.8 units	5 units
250 ml	2 units	3 units	3.75 units				

travel history is important in accessing possible exposure to viruses as hepatitis viruses are endemic in some areas of the world.

Examination

Preparation

You should begin by obtaining informed consent for the examination from the patient. The patient should be comfortable and positioned lying flat with their head resting on a single pillow to relax the abdominal muscles and facilitate abdominal palpation. Position a blanket to maintain patient dignity but remember that a full examination of the abdomen will include examination of the groins and genitalia in order not to miss important signs that can indicate life-threatening disease.

Routine

When examining the abdomen it is important to remember that there are a number of organ systems contained within it. The account below mainly outlines a schema to focus on disorders of the hepatobiliary system but the possibility of pathology in other systems (e.g. renal or gastrointestinal) must always be considered.

The examination follows the standard routine of inspection, palpation, percussion and auscultation. In patients with liver disease a lot of information can be gained from examining the limbs, face and chest and these areas must not be forgotten in the eagerness to examine the abdomen. Patients should be examined methodically and at the end of the examination the findings should be presented in the same order:

- General inspection from the end of the bed.
- Hands and arms.
- Face.
- Neck and chest.
- Abdomen.
- Groins, perineum and legs.

General inspection

After introducing yourself and positioning the patient, take a few steps back and look carefully at the patient and around the bed. If available you should look at:

- Medication.
- Dictary restriction, e.g. low salt, NBM (nil by mouth).
- Other equipment (IV cannula, urinary catheter, nasogastric tube).
- Temperature chart.

Next look at the patient but continue to resist the temptation to begin physical examination as much useful infor-

mation can be obtained from careful observation. Note the general appearance of the patient:

- Are they resting comfortably or in obvious pain? Visceral pain, such as seen in cholecystitis, might result in a restless patient; peritoneal pain, such as that caused by a perforated viscus, usually produces a still patient but inspection of the face will usually suggest that they are in pain.
- Are there features of weight loss present? Look for folds of loose skin; observe whether clothes are too big. Chronic liver disease tends to result in muscle wasting which is often obvious in the face and upper limbs.
- Is the patient alert and cooperative or are they drowsy or confused, which might suggest encephalopathy?
- Examine the colour of the patient's skin. Is there jaundice (yellow discolouration of the skin and sclera) or pigmentation (haemochromatosis may produce a 'bronze' pigmentation due to haemosiderin stimulating melanocytes to produce melanin)?

Hands and nails

Next take the patients hands and examine them carefully. Time spent examining the hands is well spent as there are many signs there that give clues to the presence of chronic liver disease. None of these signs are specific for liver disease, however, but the presence of one or more of them are suggestive.

Finger clubbing

Clubbing is swelling of the soft tissue of the end of the fingers or toes. Inspection from the side reveals a loss of the angle between the nail bed and the finger and palpation may reveal an increased sponginess of the nail bed. Eventually the distal phalanx becomes enlarged due to the soft tissue swelling. The mechanism of clubbing is uncertain but it may result from arteriovenous shunting in the lungs producing arterial desaturation that results in dilatation of the vessels of the fingertips or toes. Causes of clubbing are given in Box G.

Box G Causes of clubbing

• Abdominal	Cirrhosis, inflammatory bowel disease, coeliac disease, gastrointestinal lymphoma
• Cardiac	Congenital cyanotic heart disease, subacute bacterial endocarditis
• Respiratory	Pulmonary fibrosis, chronic pulmonary infection (e.g. bronchiectasis, abscess, empyema), cancer
• Other	Thyrotoxicosis, familial, idiopathic

Leuconychia

Leuconychia is the term given to the white discolouration of the nails seen when they opacify. There is often a rim of pink nail bed at the top of the nail. Leuconychia occurs in hypoalbuminaemia, which may be secondary to chronic liver disease, but is also seen in nephrotic syndrome and protein-losing enteropathies. The mechanism is uncertain but may reflect compression of capillary flow by extracellular fluid accumulation.

Dupuytren's contracture

Dupuytren's* contracture is a thickening of the palmar fascia that causes permanent flexion of the fingers, most often the ring finger. In the early phases it may not be visible but can be felt as a thick ridge by the examiner's thumb palpating across the patient's palm. It is often bilateral and occasionally affects the soles of the feet. If it is found in a patient with liver disease it strongly suggests alcoholism. It can also be seen in manual workers and may be idiopathic.

Palmar erythema

This is a reddening of the palms of the hands which is especially prominent over the thenar and hypothenar eminences. It is seen in chronic liver disease but also in pregnancy, thyrotoxicosis, rheumatoid arthritis and polycythaemia. The aetiology is uncertain but it may reflect raised oestrogen levels that occur due to impaired hepatic metabolism of sex hormones.

Hepatic flap

Before leaving the hands examine for the presence of a hepatic flap or asterixis. Ask the patient to stretch out their arms in front of them, extend the wrists and spread their fingers apart. Irregular jerky movements at the wrists and fingers indicate the asterixis of hepatic encephalopathy. You should examine the patient in this position for 20–30 seconds to exclude confidentally a flap. Asterixis is usually present bilaterally but the movements are not synchronous on each side. The mechanism is thought to reflect metabolic interference with the flow of joint position sense information to the brainstem. The flap is characteristic of liver failure (acute or chronic) but can also be seen in cardiac, respiratory and renal failure.

---

*Baron Guillaume Dupuytren (1799–1835), French surgeon.

Arms

Examination of the patient with suspected liver disease requires a thorough inspection of the arms as many clues to the presence of liver disease may be found there. Again, these are not specific but their presence can be a strong indicator of liver pathology.

Spider naevi

Spider naevi are abnormal vessels usually found on the skin in the area drained by the superior vena cava (i.e. the arms, head and neck, and upper chest wall), the reason for this distribution is not known. They consist of a central arteriole with small vessels radiating out from it resembling spiders' legs. Pressure applied at the central arteriole causes the entire lesion to blanch. They are usually a few millimetres in size but occasionally can be up to a centimetre. One or two may be seen in healthy individuals but the presence of more than two is abnormal. They are sometimes seen in the latter stages of pregnancy or in women on the contraceptive pill raising the suggestion that they are caused by oestrogen-mediated dilatation on arterioles. They occasionally bleed but the main concern they cause the patient is usually cosmetic.

Bruising

Examination of the arms of a patient with liver disease frequently reveals bruising (ecchymoses) reflecting the clotting abnormalities seen in liver disease. These may be spontaneous or occur at the site of previous venepuncture or intravenous cannulation.

Petechiae

Pin-sized bruises may also be present and usually suggest thrombocytopenia. This may be caused by platelet sequestration and destruction in an enlarged spleen in portal hypertension or bone marrow depression, which is often a feature of chronic alcohol consumption.

Scratch marks

Patients with obstructive jaundice or cholestasis may be troubled by severe itch (pruritus). This sensation is often so intense that patients cannot resist the urge to itch and can frequently scratch until they bleed leaving grazes and marks on their skin.

Muscle wasting

Before leaving the upper limbs carefully inspect them for evidence of loss of muscle bulk, which is often seen in severe chronic liver disease or in a patient with underlying malignancy.

Face
Jaundice
Examine the sclera carefully for jaundice as this is often the only site that it can be detected clinically. Jaundice is the only condition to cause yellow sclera, so if the skin is yellow but not the sclerae then a diagnosis other than jaundice should be sought (e.g. carotenaemia).

Kayser–Fleischer rings
These are brownish green rings at the periphery of the cornea, tending to affect the upper pole more than the lower. They are due to deposits of excess copper in Descemet's membrane of the cornea. They are difficult to see, especially in dark eyed individuals, and a slit-lamp examination is often necessary to demonstrate them. They are most commonly associated with Wilson's disease, a copper storage disease that causes cirrhosis and neurological symptoms, but can also be seen in patients with other cholestatic liver diseases. They are much loved in picture books and exams but very rarely seen in clinical practice.

Xanthelasma
These yellowish plaques in the subcutaneous tissues in the periorbital region are due to deposits of lipids. They may indicate chronic hypercholesterolaemia. They can be seen in patients with cholestasis and are particularly common in patients with primary biliary cirrhosis.

Parotid enlargement
Palpate the cheeks to examine for enlargement of the parotid glands. This can be seen in alcoholism, which causes fatty infiltration of the gland.

Hepatic fetor
Examine the mouth closely and note the presence of fetor hepaticus, a rather sweet smell of the breath which is present with severe hepatocellular dysfunction. It is important to familiarise yourself with this smell since detection of its presence in a patient with a coma of otherwise unknown cause can be a very helpful clue to the diagnosis of hepatic encephalopathy.

Neck and chest
Palpate the cervical lymph nodes, which can be involved in advanced intra-abdominal malignancy. Examine the chest wall for spider naevi and for the presence of gynaecomastia in males. Enlargement of the breast tissue may occur in cirrhosis, particularly alcoholic cirrhosis, and is thought to reflect alteration in the oestrogen:testosterone ratio. Spironolactone, used to treat ascites in cirrhosis and other conditions, is another cause of gynaecomastia, as are digoxin and cimetidine.

Abdomen
Now attention can be turned to the abdomen itself.

Inspection
Look for abdominal scars that may indicate previous surgery or trauma. Note the presence of generalised abdominal distension that could reflect ascites but will need to be differentiated from fat, flatus, faeces, organomegaly and tumours. Localised swellings may indicate a tumour mass, enlargement of one of the abdominal or pelvic organs or a hernia.

In a patient with liver disease and portal hypertension, prominent veins may be obvious on the abdominal wall. Blood flows through portosystemic anastomoses into the umbilical veins, which become engorged and distended. The direction of flow is away from the umbilicus. This sign is called a caput Medusae (head of Medusa), likening the appearance to the mythical Medusa's hair after it had been turned into snakes. This needs to be differentiated from venous engorgement secondary to inferior vena cava obstruction when the direction of flow in the engorged veins is upward towards the heart.

Palpation
This part of the examination often reveals the most information but in order to achieve this it is vital that the patient is comfortable and the abdominal muscles are relaxed. Ask the patient if any area is painful before you start and examine this area last. Encourage the patient to breathe gently throughout the examination and to inform you if there is any tenderness.

The abdomen is divided into nine regions (Fig. O) and each area should be palpated with the palmar surface of the fingers. Begin with light pressure in each region, noting the presence of any tenderness or lumps in each region. Next perform firmer palpation to detect deeper masses, taking care to avoid the tender areas until the end of the examination. Note the presence of guarding, resistance to palpation that occurs due to contraction of the abdominal muscles. This may be voluntary due to anxiety or tenderness; involuntary guarding suggests peritonitis.

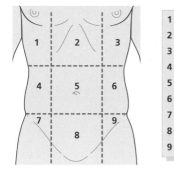

1	Right hypochondrium
2	Epigastrium
3	Left hypochondrium
4	Right lumbar region
5	Umbilical region
6	Left lumbar region
7	Right iliac fossa
8	Suprapubic region
9	Left iliac fossa

Figure O Regions of the abdomen.

After superficial and deep palpation, the presence of organomegaly should be specifically sought.

Hepatomegaly

An enlarged liver can often be palpated in the abdomen below the right costal margin. The examining hand should be held parallel to the costal margin with the lateral margin of the forefinger towards the lowest rib. Ask the patient to breathe in and out slowly and keeping your hand still feel for the liver edge as it descends in inspiration. It is important to begin examining in the right iliac fossa so as not to miss the edge of a massively enlarged liver. With each expiration, advance the hand 1 or 2 cm closer to the right costal margin. This examination should continue into the epigastrium as it is not uncommon for the left lobe of the liver to be palpable to the left of the midline in cirrhosis. If the liver edge is felt examine its surface for tenderness and to determine whether the liver is hard or soft, regular or irregular, and whether it is pulsatile.

There are many causes of an enlarged liver (Box H). It is important to remember that liver disease can also result in a small liver that may not be palpable. For example, in cirrhosis the fibrous scarring usually results in a small shrunken liver, and in acute liver necrosis the liver shrinks rapidly due to hepatocyte death.

The gallbladder

The gallbladder lies below the right costal margin where this crosses the lateral border of the rectus muscles. It is not usually palpable in health but if it is enlarged may be felt as a focal rounded mass that moves down on inspiration. In cholecystitis, palpation at the costal margin

causes severe pain when the inflamed gallbladder presses on the examiner's hand (Murphy's sign[†]).

The causes of an enlarged gallbladder are listed in Box I. It is important to remember Courvoisier's law,[‡] which states that an enlarged gallbladder in a patient with jaundice is unlikely to be due to gallstones as this situation usually results in a chronically inflamed and fibrotic gallbladder incapable of enlargement. In a jaundiced patient, a palpable gallbladder is more likely to be caused by carcinoma of the head of the pancreas or lower biliary

---

Box H Causes of hepatomegaly

Common causes
- Alcohol-related liver disease with fatty infiltration
- Right heart failure
- Metastases
- Hepatitis
- Fatty liver disease (e.g. secondary to diabetes and the metabolic syndrome)

Other causes
- Malignancy (hepatocellular carcinoma, myeloproliferative disorders, lymphoproliferative disorders)
- Infections (infectious mononucleosis, malaria, HIV, hepatic abscesses, hydatid disease)
- Haemochromatosis
- Infiltration (e.g. amyloid)
- Biliary obstruction

Tender liver
- Hepatitis
- Rapid enlargement (right heart failure, Budd–Chiari syndrome*)
- Hepatic abscesses

Pulsatile liver
- Tricuspid regurgitation
- Vascular abnormalities
- Hepatocellular carcinoma

Firm, irregular liver
- Cirrhosis
- Metastatic disease

*George Budd (1808–1882), Professor of medicine, King's College Hospital, London. Hans Chiari (1851–1916), Professor of pathology, Prague.

[†]John Murphy (1857–1916), American surgeon.
[‡]Ludwig Courvoisier (1843–1918), Professor of surgery, Switzerland.

> ### Box I Causes of gallbladder enlargement
>
> **With jaundice**
> - Carcinoma of the head of the pancreas
> - Carcinoma of the ampulla of Vater
> - Gallstone formed in the common bile duct in the absence of gallbladder stones
>
> **Without jaundice**
> - Empyema or mucocoele of the gallbladder
> - Carcinoma of the gallbladder
> - Acute cholecystitis

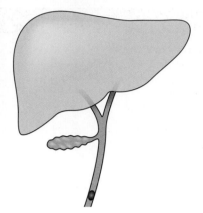

(a) Obstructive jaundice due to a gallstone is usually associated with a thickened contracted gallbladder

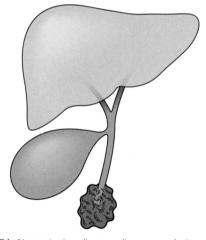

(b) Obstructive jaundice to malignancy results in a distended gallbladder which may be palpable

Figure P Courvoisier's law.

tree, resulting in biliary obstruction (Fig. P). The reverse is not necessarily true however, an impalpable bladder in a jaundiced patient may be due to gallstones but other causes are also possible since it is common for a gallbladder to be dilated but impalpable.

Splenomegaly

An enlarged spleen cannot usually be detected clinically until it is about twice its normal size. In the early stages of enlargement, the spleen can be felt just below the left costal margin towards its lateral margin. Further enlargement causes it to project inferiorly and medially. Examination for an enlarged spleen should therefore begin in the right iliac fossa so as not to miss a massively enlarged spleen. Begin with the hand flat on the abdomen with the index finger parallel to the left costal margin. Keeping the hand still ask the patient to breathe in and feel for the spleen tip descending in inspiration. In expiration advance the examining hand towards the left costal margin. Palpation of a slightly enlarged spleen can be helped by using a two-handed approach. As the right hand approaches the costal margin use the left hand to compress firmly posterolaterally over the lower rib cage so as to remove the tension in the abdominal wall. If the spleen is not palpable, the patient should be rolled onto their right side towards the examiner and palpation using the two-handed technique repeated. The causes of splenomegaly are given in Box J and hepatosplenomegaly in Box K.

Other organs

If you are asked to examine the abdomen then an attempt to palpate the kidneys must be made. Even if hepatobiliary disease is suspected it is necessary to consider a renal mass in the differential diagnosis of a right or left sub-

costal mass. Kidneys are best felt by bimanual palpation with the patient lying flat on his or her back. For the right kidney place the left hand underneath the patient's back with the palm in the right loin and the flexing fingers in the renal angle. Press this hand forward whilst the right hand presses down on the anterior abdomen above it. With this technique, called balloting, the kidney may be felt between the two hands. The opposite hands are used for the left kidney. Box L outlines the features that differentiate a kidney from a spleen.

Other masses may be palpable on abdominal examination. If a mass is found then it should be fully characterised asking the following questions:

Box J Causes of splenomegaly

Massive splenomegaly
- Haematological (myelofibrosis, chronic myeloid leukaemia, primary lymphoma of the spleen)
- Portal hypertension
- Infection (malaria, Kala azar)

Moderate splenomegaly
- The above causes
- Haematological malignancy (e.g. lymphoma, leukaemia)
- Thalassaemia
- Storage disorders (e.g. Gaucher's disease)

Small splenomegaly
- The above causes
- Other myeloproliferative disorders (essential thrombocytosis, polycythaemia rubra vera)
- Haemolytic anaemia
- Connective tissue disorders (e.g. rheumatoid arthritis, systemic lupus erythematosus, polyarteritis nodosa)
- Infection: bacterial (e.g. infective endocarditis, tuberculosis); viral (e.g. Epstein–Barr virus, viral hepatitis); protozoa (e.g. malaria)
- Infiltration (e.g. amyloid, sarcoid)

Box K Causes of hepatosplenomegaly

- Chronic liver disease with portal hypertension
- Infection (e.g. acute viral hepatitis)
- Haematological disease (e.g. myeloproliferative disease, lymphoma, leukaemia, pernicious anaemia, sickle cell anaemia)
- Connective tissue disorder (e.g. systemic lupus erythematosus)
- Infiltration (e.g. amyloid, sarcoid)
- Thyrotoxicosis
- Acromegaly

- What is the site of the mass? State the region of the abdomen involved using Fig. O.
- Is it possible to palpate above it?
- What is its size and shape?
- Is the surface smooth or irregular?
- Is the edge regular or irregular?
- What is the consistency (e.g. hard or soft)?
- Is the mass mobile? Does it move on inspiration?
- Is it pulsatile?
- Is there any tenderness?

Box L Differences between a spleen and kidney on clinical examination

- The upper border of the spleen cannot be palpated as it lies above the costal margin. The upper border of the kidney can be palpated
- The spleen has a notch which can be palpated. The kidney does not have a notch
- The kidney is ballottable between the two examining hands because of its retroperitoneal location. The spleen is not usually ballottable
- The spleen moves inferomedially towards the right iliac fossa on inspiration whereas the left kidney moves inferiorly towards the left iliac fossa
- Percussion over the spleen is usually dull but percussion over the kidney is resonant as it lies underneath gas-filled bowel

Percussion

Abdominal percussion is performed to define the size and nature of organs and masses, to find out whether distension is due to gas, free fluid (ascites), encased fluid (e.g. a cyst) or a solid mass and to elicit tenderness in a patient with peritonitis.

Liver

The liver borders should be percussed to determine the total liver span. Percuss down the chest along the midclavicular line noting where the percussion note changes from resonant to dull, normally level with the sixth rib. The measurement from this point to the palpable liver edge gives the liver span, usually less than 12 cm in health. If the liver edge is palpable, assessing the liver span is important to determine whether the liver is enlarged or merely displaced downwards, for example by overinflated emphysematous lungs. With experience it is also possible to define a small, shrunken cirrhotic liver by percussion.

Spleen

Percussion is not a particularly helpful method of detecting an enlarged spleen but can sometimes be helpful if it is doubtful whether the tip can be felt.

Ascites

Accumulation of fluid within the peritoneum may be suspected by inspection and palpation but must be confirmed by percussion. Percussion over the abdomen normally produces a resonant note due to air within the gastrointestinal tract. If peritoneal fluid (ascites) is present the percussion note becomes dull. The liquid gravitates to the dependent part of the abdomen, thus in the supine patient there is dullness in the flanks and this dullness shifts when the patient is rotated onto their side. This phenomenon is referred to as shifting dullness.

When examining for ascites place the left hand on the abdomen over the midline with the fingers of the left hand pointing to the feet. Strike the middle phalanyx of the left middle finger with the tip of the right middle finger. Percuss from the resonant centre of the abdomen into the left flank until the percussion note becomes dull. Keep the left hand in place and ask the patient to roll onto their right side. Pause for a few seconds to allow the fluid to move then repeat percussion. If the percussion note has become resonant and percussion back towards the umbilicus re-establishes a dull note, ascites is suggested. Occasionally a large ovarian cyst or fluid within dilated bowel in small intestinal obstruction can cause confusion.

In massive ascites, a *fluid thrill* may be detectable although this is not examined for routinely. Ask an assistant to place a hand firmly on the centre of the abdomen. Flick the side of the abdominal wall and feel for a pulsation (thrill) with the other hand placed on the other side of the abdomen. An additional useful technique when there is significant ascites is *dipping* over the upper abdomen to determine if the liver or spleen is enlarged. Place the hand flat on the abdomen and flex the fingers at the metacarpophalangeal joints rapidly to displace underlying fluid. The rapid displacement of fluid allows the fingers to reach an organ or mass covered in ascites.

Causes of ascites are given in Box M.

Auscultation

Many abdominal sounds have been described in patients with liver disease but in general it is rare for auscultation to be very contributory to the examination of the hepatobiliary system. It must be performed as part of the complete abdominal examination, however, and is essential so as not to miss vital signs that can suggest bowel obstruction or perforation.

Using the diaphragm of the stethoscope, listen over the abdomen for the presence and character of bowel sounds, friction rubs, arterial bruits and venous hums. If the liver is enlarged it is important to listen over its surface. A friction rub is a grating sound heard when the patient breathes; it is produced by inflammation in the liver

---

Box M Causes of ascites

- Cirrhosis
- Congestive cardiac failure
- Intra-abdominal malignancy (e.g. gastrointestinal, gynaecological)
- Pancreatitis
- Infection (e.g. pyogenic, tuberculosis)
- Budd–Chiari syndrome
- Meig's syndrome*
- Nephrotic syndrome
- Protein-losing enteropathy
- Hypothyroidism

*Joe Vincent Meigs (Professor of gynaecology, Harvard 1942–55) described a syndrome of fibroma of the ovary with ascites and hydrothorax.

---

capsule (e.g. by a liver tumour, a hepatic infarct, a recent liver biopsy or the very rare Fitz-Hugh–Curtis syndrome[†] when a perihepatitis complicates pelvic inflammatory disease). Arterial systolic bruits are occasionally heard over the liver in hepatocellular carcinoma, acute alcoholic hepatitis or with an arteriovenous malformation. More commonly, arterial bruits are due to stenoses in the aorta, mesenteric or renal arteries. Rarely, a venous hum can be heard between the xiphisternum and umbilicus due to turbulence in the collateral circulation in portal hypertension.

Further examination

To complete the examination of the abdominal system it is essential to examine the hernia orifices, the external genitalia and perform a rectal examination (Box N). Examine the legs for pitting oedema.

On finishing your examination thank the patient, help them back into their clothing and ensure that they are left in a comfortable position. A summary of the clinical examination of a patient with suspected liver disease is given in Box O.

Putting it all together

Once the history and examination findings have been recorded the information needs to be analysed in order to:

[†]Thomas Fitz-Hugh (1894–1963), haematologist, Pennsylvania. Arthur Curtis (1881–1955), Professor of obstetrics and gynaecology, Chicago.

> **Box N Relevance of the rectal examination in liver disease**
>
> - Pale stools: obstructive jaundice/cholestasis
> - Melaena: upper gastrointestinal bleeding (may identify the cause of encephalopathy in someone presenting in a coma)
> - Constipation: may exacerbate encephalopathy
> - Steatorrhoea: malabsorption which may be a feature of cholestasis

- Consider the differential diagnosis. In straightforward cases a single provisional diagnosis may be evident. In others a number of possible diagnoses may need to be considered.
- Create a problem list. In some complicated cases it may be necessary to create a problem list considering new complaints, co-morbidities and social circumstances.
- Create a strategy for investigation.
- Develop a treatment plan.
- Arrange follow-up.

A plan for further review of the patient needs to be documented. If seen in the GP surgery or outpatient clinic this may be to be reviewed again when the results of investigations are available or to contact the patient to let them know the investigation results. A patient attending the emergency department may need to be admitted or discharged with investigations organised as an outpatient.

Investigations performed in hepatology
Blood tests
Blood investigations are an important aspect in managing patients with liver disease and are able to give insight into hepatic damage, hepatic function, aetiology of disease and prognosis.

Liver function tests
The term 'liver function tests' (LFTs) is a misnomer as these tests are not optimal measures of hepatic function (albumin and coagulation are more useful 'functional' tests). Nonetheless LFTS can alert clinicians to the possibility of underlying hepatic injury. Moreover, the pattern of abnormality in LFTS is often more helpful in clinical practice than individual test results. The following are the most commonly used LFTs:

- *Alanine aminotransferase (ALT)*: This is an enzyme that catalyses the conversion of alanine to pyruvate. It is present is high concentrations within hepatocytes so elevated levels suggest hepatocyte damage/necrosis.
- *Aspartate aminotransferase (AST)*: AST is located in the mitochondrial membrane in hepatocytes but is also contained in erythrocytes, myocardium and skeletal muscle. In the context of liver disease it reflects hepatocellular necrosis. Generally, hepatitis results in a similar pattern of elevation in both AST and ALT. An elevated AST:ALT ratio, however, can indicate alcoholic liver disease or signify liver fibrosis in the context of non-alcoholic liver disease.
- *Alkaline phosphatase (ALP)*: A number of isoenzymes of ALP exist including bone, intestine, placenta and liver. An elevation in the liver ALP isoform can be indicative of biliary disease or cholestasis (intrahepatic or extrahepatic).
- *Gamma glutamyl transferase (γ-GT)*: This can be raised in a number of liver conditions including alcoholic liver disease, cholestasis and liver fibrosis. An elevated γ-GT can be helpful in the context of a raised ALP in suggesting a hepatic origin for the ALP.
- *Bilirubin*: This is elevated in haemolysis, cholestasis or impaired hepatic function. Distinguishing unconjugated (indirect) bilirubin from conjugated (direct) bilirubin can be useful in some cases.

Synthetic function
Prolongation of the prothombin time (PT) can imply significant liver disease as the liver is incapable of synthesising normal coagulation factors. It can also occur in the presence of cholestasis or malnutrition due to interruption of gastrointestinal vitamin K absorption (a fat-soluble vitamin dependent on bile salts for absorption). Administration of intravenous vitamin K will correct for any reduced absorption (due to biliary disease or malnutrition) but will not correct abnormalities related to hepatic synthesis.

Reduced serum albumin is a feature of chronic liver disease and a falling albumin has prognostic significance. It should be noted that any major insult causing a stress response (e.g. surgery, sepsis, injury, etc.) will lead to an acute reduction in albumin production.

Renal function and electrolytes
Low urea and creatinine concentrations in liver disease reflect the reduced muscle mass that accompanies cirrhosis. Therefore absolute values of creatinine may falsely

Box O OSCE checklist for abdominal examination focusing on chronic liver disease

Introduction

Introduces self (name and position)	1 mark
Explains procedure to the patient	1 mark
Asks consent to examine the patient	1 mark
Washes hands	1 mark
Positions patient lying flat with one pillow and ensures patient is comfortable	1 mark

General examination

Observes the patient from the end of the bed	1 mark
Comments on equipment and material around the patient	1 mark

Hands

Examines the patient correctly for the presence or absence of:

Clubbing	1 mark
Leuconychia	1 mark
Palmar erythema	1 mark
Dupuytren's contracture	1 mark
Hepatic asterixis	1 mark

Upper body and face

Comments on the presence or absence of:

Spider naevi	1 mark
Bruising/petechiae	1 mark
Muscle wasting	1 mark
Gynaecomastia	1 mark
Examines the eyes for jaundice	1 mark
Examines the parotids, cervical and axillary lymph nodes	1 mark

Abdomen

Observes the abdomen noting scars, distension and prominent veins	1 mark
Performs light palpation with care noting any masses or areas of tenderness	1 mark
Performs deep palpation carefully	1 mark
Examines correctly for hepatomegaly starting in the right iliac fossa and examining in inspiration. If enlarged, examines the liver edge and surface	2 marks
Examines correctly for splenomegaly including rolling the patient on their right side and bimanually palpating under the costal margin in inspiration	2 marks
Examines for enlarged kidneys	1 mark
Percusses over the liver to determine liver span	1 mark
Percusses over the rest of the abdomen defining any masses or organomegaly	1 mark
Percusses correctly for ascites including rolling the patient	2 marks
Auscultates the abdomen noting the presence and character of bowel sounds, presence of bruits and listens over the liver	1 mark
Offers to examine the hernia orifices, external genitalia and perform a rectal examination	1 mark

Summing it up

Comments correctly on findings	2 marks
Summarises examination findings correctly	3 marks
Gives a differential diagnosis	3 marks

Total **40 marks**

Table H Tests for screening liver disease.

Test	Aetiology	Notes
Hepatitis C antibody	Hepatitis C	If positive, the polymerase chain reaction (PCR) will clarify if there is active HCV viraemia
Hepatitis B surface antigen	Hepatitis B	Surface antigen positivity needs further investigation by HBV DNA ± liver biopsy
Immunoglobulins	Autoimmune hepatitis	Elevated immunoglobulins are typical of this disorder
Autoimmune profile	Autoimmune hepatitis and primary biliary cirrhosis	Antibodies commonly tested are antinuclear antibody (ANA), smooth muscle antibody (SMA), anti-liver kidney microsomal antibodies (LKMs) and antimitochondrial antibodies (AMAs)
Ferritin (transferrin saturation)	Haemochromatosis	Iron studies can be difficult to interpret in acute hepatitis and ferritin is elevated in any acute phase response. Testing for genetic mutations (e.g. C282Y) may be useful
Alpha-1 antitrypsin level and phenotype	Alpha-1 antitrypsin deficiency	The pathology in the liver differs to lung disease and is a result of abnormal protein accumulating within hepatocytes
Caeruloplasmin	Wilson's disease	A normal caeruloplasmin does not exclude Wilson's disease and if there is clinical suspicion further investigation including a penicillamine challenge and liver biopsy may be warranted

HBV, hepatitis B virus; HCV, hepatitis C virus.

reassure and glomerular filtration rates or the relative change in creatinine may be a better indicator of renal function. It is particularly important to monitor renal function in decompensated cirrhosis as early diagnosis of renal dysfunction, with instigation of treatment, may reverse the condition.

In advanced cirrhosis, total body overload of salt and water occurs; body water retention exceeds sodium retention resulting in hyponatraemia. Secondary hyperaldosteronism is common in cirrhosis and results in hypokalaemia. Other electrolyte disturbances such as hypophosphataemia, hypomagnesaemia and reduced serum selenium are not uncommon in patients with advanced liver disease. These may require correction by intravenous therapy to prevent refeeding syndrome when liver disease patients are hospitalised.

Full blood count
A pancytopenia (low white blood cell count, haemoglobin and platelet count) in cirrhosis occurs as a result of portal hypertension causing pooling of blood in the splanchnic circulation. Certain aetiological agents (e.g.

alcohol) can also cause bone marrow suppression. The production of the hormone thrombopoietin, involved in the synthesis of platelets, is reduced in advanced liver disease and this will also contribute to the thrombocytopenia. Haemolysis is associated with certain aetiologies of liver disease (e.g. autoimmune hepatitis, Zieve's syndrome* and Wilson's disease).

Tests for the aetiology of liver disease
Liver disease is often asymptomatic and therefore blood tests are an important diagnostic tool in determining the aetiology of the disease. The chronic liver disease screen is a useful set of investigations in patients presenting with chronically deranged liver function tests (Table H).

Tumour markers
The common tumour markers used in liver disease are α-fetoprotein (AFP) and CA19-9:

---

*Zieve's syndrome is a combination of alcoholic liver disease, haemolytic anaemia and hypertriglyceridaemia.

• AFP is produced by regenerating hepatocytes and therefore can be raised in chronic liver disease and cirrhosis *per se*. A single AFP reading has limitations but a persistently elevated AFP on follow-up is a strong indicator of hepatocellular carcinoma (HCC).

• CA19-9 is a commonly used tumour marker for cholangiocarcinoma. The sensitivity and specificity of the test is not optimal; for example, any cause of cholestasis or cholangitis may elevate the CA19-9. Therefore it can be rarely used to diagnose cholangiocarcinoma without support from radiological imaging or biopsy.

• CA125 can be elevated in any cause of ascites; this needs to be considered in the context of investigating ovarian disease and coexisting liver disease.

Imaging

Hepatobiliary radiology is complex and close liaison with a hepatobiliary radiologist to decide on appropriate investigation and to aid interpretation in the correct clinical context is an important interface in clinical hepatology.

Ultrasound

Ultrasound (US) is a relatively inexpensive, non-invasive method of assessing the biliary system, the size and echotexture of the liver, vascular patency and in detecting space-occupying lesions within the liver (Fig. Q). It is a useful first-line imaging investigation for the jaundiced patient.

• Dilated intrahepatic bile ducts on US suggest an obstructive cause such as gallstones in the common bile duct, a pancreatic carcinoma or cholangiocarcinoma.

• Gallstones can easily be seen in the gallbladder using US. Stones in the common bile duct are more difficult to visualise by US and often require more specialist investigations such as magnetic resonance cholangiopancreatography (MRCP), computed tomography (CT) and endoscopic retrograde cholangiopancreatography (ERCP).

• The cirrhotic liver may be enlarged (e.g. in non-alcoholic steatohepatitis), normal or reduced in size. The echopattern of the liver is frequently described as coarse (increased irregular echogenicity) in cirrhosis and the margin of the liver may be irregular.

• The presence of ascites and splenomegaly on US examination in patients with liver disease is strongly suggestive of cirrhosis (the main differential is portal vein thrombosis).

• Doppler ultrasound provides a technique to measure blood flow in the portal vein, hepatic artery and hepatic veins. It measures the frequency differences between the US signal emitted from the transducer and returned from the vessel; this generates direction and velocity of blood flow. The major vascular changes seen in cirrhosis reflect underlying portal hypertension. They include the reversal of portal vein blood from hepatopetal to hepatofugal, flattening of the Doppler waveform in hepatic veins, and enlargement of the portal vein to greater than 15 mm.

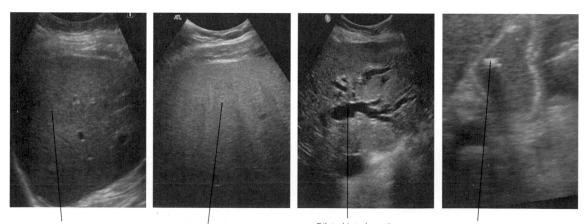

Normal hepatic parenchyma

Bright echotexture consistent with fatty infiltration

Dilated intrahepatic bile ducts

Gallstone casting an acoustic shadow

Figure Q Liver ultrasound examination.

PART 1: BASICS

• Ultrasound is used as a screening tool to detect HCC on the background of cirrhosis. Isolated nodules, larger than 2 cm, are detected with a good sensitivity but a lower specificity. The performance of US in the presence of diffuse malignancy is poor. Confirmation of US findings of HCC are required by cross-sectional imaging (CT or magnetic resonance imaging (MRI)).

Computed tomography

• CT provides cross-sectional anatomy of the liver. With the advent of multislice CT scanning detailed information about space-occupying lesions can be gleaned with very short acquisition times.

• Helical CT can also utilise vascular anomalies of lesions by obtaining images in the arterial, portal venous phase and delayed phase (triple phase). For example HCC will typically have a brisk enhancement during the arterial phase (Fig. R) but appears hypodense during the delayed phase (rapid washout).

• Direct catheterisation of the superior mesenteric artery and hepatic artery can also be used in combination with CT to improve diagnostic accuracy. Therefore, CT in isolation or combination with arteriography is able to provide a vascular 'road map' highlighting the blood supply of lesions or vascular anomalies.

• CT is not the ideal modality to assess liver parenchyma. However, in certain aetiologies changes in the density of liver parenchyma can be pronounced; e.g. increased density in haemochromatosis and decreased density in fatty infiltration.

Magnetic resonance imaging

More detailed images of liver parenchyma can be obtained by MRI compared to CT; furthermore patients are not subjected to ionising radiation. The major disadvantage is the availability of equipment and time required to acquire the images.

• MRI can be useful in diagnosing benign conditions such as haemangiomas, focal nodular hyperplasia and adenomas. The use of contrast agents such as lipiodol, gadolinium and superparamagnetic contrast agents (e.g. resovist) are often utilised to separate benign lesions from HCC.

• MRI has been used to assess hepatic iron concentration.

• Magnetic resonance (MR) angiography (useful in assessing vasculature) and MR spectroscopy (with a role in assessing hepatic steatosis) are emerging areas of MRI.

MRCP and ERCP

• MRCP is a non-invasive method of assessing the pancreatic and biliary tree. With improving hardware and technical expertise it represents the preferred modality for the diagnosis of biliary gallstones (Fig. S(a)) in comparison to more invasive ERCP. In addition, it is useful

Hepatocellular carcinoma demonstrating arterial phase enhancement

Aorta (bright due to infusion of contrast in the arterial phase)

Spleen

Figure R CT scan of the abdomen demonstrating hepatocellular carcinoma within the liver.

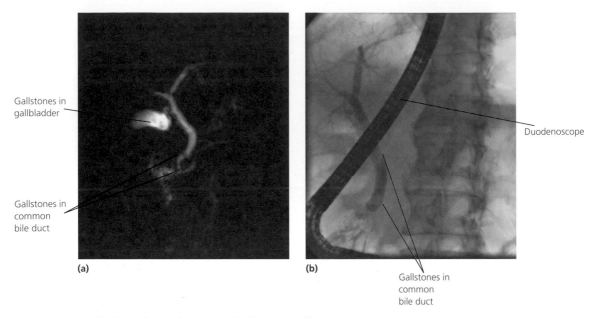

Gallstones in gallbladder

Gallstones in common bile duct

Duodenoscope

Gallstones in common bile duct

(a) (b)

Figure S Common bile duct gallstones demonstrated by (a) MRCP and (b) ERCP.

in the diagnosis of conditions such as biliary strictures, primary sclerosing cholangitis, pancreatic divisum and cholangicarcinoma.

• ERCP is largely a therapeutic modality in modern-day practice. The specially designed endoscope has a side viewer allowing visualisation and cannulation of the biliary and pancreatic tree (Fig. S(b)). For gallstone disease, it allows the removal of gallstones and dissection of the ampulla of Vater (sphincterotomy). ERCP is also used to place stents across strictures of the pancreatic and biliary duct. The complications of ERCP include bleeding, pancreatitis and perforation of the bowel so considered thought should be given before undertaking the procedure.

Miscellaneous procedures

• Arteriography can be useful for detailed characterisation of hepatic vasculature (Fig. T). In addition it may aid the diagnosis of HCC, find the source of haemorrhage within the liver and be part of therapy in HCC (transarterial chemoembolisation is when chemotherapy agents are delivered locally to the HCC and the feeding blood vessel to the tumour is simultaneously embolised).

• Percutaneous transhepatic cholangiography (PTC) is utilised by interventional radiologists to access the

biliary tree (Fig. U). It is often required in high strictures (e.g. hilar strictures) when access is not possible by ERCP.

• Endoscopic ultrasound (EUS) has become an important tool in hepatobiliary disease. In addition to staging disease (e.g. pancreatic carcinoma), it is used to obtain tissue for histological confirmation. In the appropriate hands it is superior to MRCP for diagnosing cholelithiasis in the common bile duct and has an emerging role in the drainage of pancreatic pseudocysts, coeliac nerve plexus blocks in chronic pancreatitis and assessing submucosal gastric varices.

Histology and liver biopsy

Histological analysis is an important diagnostic tool for assessing liver disease. The method for obtaining a liver biopsy can vary from the transabdominal approach, transjugular approach, laparoscopic approach and open approach at operation or postmortem. The choice of route will depend on factors such as body habitus, clotting abnormalities, presence of ascites, available expertise and quantity of specimen required. Contraindications for the transabdominal approach are shown in Box P. The biopsy delineates aetiology (e.g. viral hepatitis, alcoholic liver disease, metabolic liver disease, etc.), severity

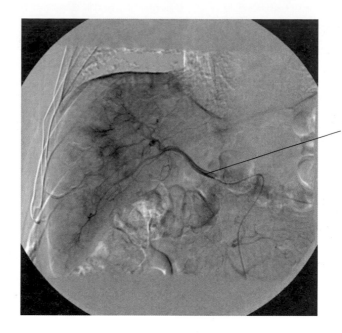

Catheter in the
hepatic artery

Figure T Hepatic arteriography.

Dilated intrahepatic biliary system

Decompressed biliary system

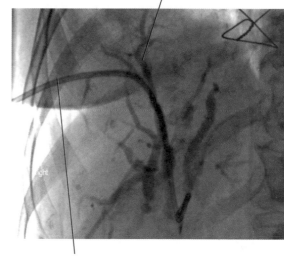

Right

ight

Percutaneous needle directly puncturing
an intrahepatic biliary radicle

Percutaneously inserted biliary drain

(a)

(b)

Figure U (a) Percutaneous transhepatic cholangiography demonstrating an obstructed biliary system. (b) The same patient after the insertion of a biliary drain.

of disease (early fibrosis or cirrhosis) and specific pathological entities (e.g. steatosis or necroinflammation in non-alcoholic fatty liver disease).

Liver biopsy does have its limitations and some have questioned whether it truly represents a 'gold standard' reference test. In large studies of patients undergoing biopsy, pain has been reported in 20% and severe complications reported in 0.57%. Sampling error exists, which is unsurprising considering the average biopsy specimen represents 1/50 000th of the organ. Interpretation of the biopsy is open both to intra- and interobserver error.

Box P Contraindications to percutaneous liver biopsy

• Coagulopathy	Biopsy not recommended if INR >1.4 or platelets <60 × 10⁹/L
• Dilated intrahepatic biliary system	Risk of bleeding into the biliary system (haemobilia)
• Marked ascites	Risk of uncontrolled bleeding into the ascites
• Cystic lesions	Risk of bleeding into cyst. Inadvertent biopsy of a hydatid cyst may result in anaphylaxis
• Severe emphysema	Risk of pneumothorax or bullous puncture leading to critical respiratory compromise
• Uncooperative patient	Patient needs to hold their breath during biopsy therefore cooperation is required
• Amyloidosis*	Increased risk of haemorrhage
• Bacterial cholangitis*	Risk of inducing peritonitis and septic shock

*Relative contraindications.

Non-invasive markers of liver fibrosis

The liver biopsy, when performed and analysed by specialists, represents a very useful tool to define aetiology and delineate specific pathology including steatosis, necroinflammation and fibrosis. However, the rising prevalence of liver disease in association with patient choice, ethical implications of an invasive diagnostic test and economic considerations have led to the development of non-invasive tests of liver fibrosis. Hitherto, these have been utilised in clinical research but they are starting to emerge in clinical practice. The tests can be divided into three broad areas:

1 Serum panel marker tests using routine clinical parameters (e.g. platelet count, AST : ALT ratio and albumin) or markers of fibrogenesis (e.g. hyaluronic acid, metalloproteases, serum type III procollagen peptide (PIII NP), etc.) or a combination.

2 Imaging modalities such as fibroscan (which measures the speed of a propagated wave across the liver using a specially adapted ultrasound device) and variants of MRI (e.g. MR spectroscopy and MR elastography).

3 High through put 'omics' technologies (e.g. proteomics).

Case 1   A 19-year-old man presenting with jaundice

Mr John Farrelly is a 19-year-old student who presents with a short history of abdominal discomfort and jaundice. He has associated symptoms of fatigue, decreased appetite and myalgia. You have been asked to review him in the jaundice clinic.

What is the differential diagnosis for his jaundice?

Jaundice can be classified into:

1 Prehepatic jaundice (e.g. haemolysis).
2 Hepatocellular jaundice (e.g. hepatitis).
3 Posthepatic jaundice (e.g. obstruction of the biliary tree).

What additional questions would be helpful in your routine history?

• *How long has he had these symptoms?* An assessment of the chronology of his symptoms should be made to try to determine whether this is an acute or chronic process. In doing so it is important to recognise that liver disease can frequently be asymptomatic for months or years prior to presentation; however, a history of vague symptoms such as tiredness or anorexia might suggest a chronic process.

• *Has he had a similar episode before?* A history of becoming jaundiced with previous viral illnesses might suggest a diagnosis of Gilbert's syndrome. Alternatively, it might represent a rarer cause of jaundice such as haemolytic anaemia or benign, recurrent intrahepatic cholestasis (BRIC), an autosomally recessive disorder characterised by intermittent attacks of cholestasis that spontaneously resolve.

• *What are the colour of his stools and urine?* Dark urine and pale stools suggests an obstructive or cholestatic picture. The presence of these changes does not differentiate between intrahepatic and extrahepatic biliary obstruction, however, but they do differentiate from a prehepatic cause of jaundice.

• *What is the nature of his pain?* Pain of biliary origin (severe, right upper quadrant pain in a band) may raise the suspicion of an obstructive picture secondary to gallstones. Pain of acute hepatitis is usually not severe but more of a dull ache over the liver.

• *Is there a history of travel?* Acute viral hepatitis may present with jaundice. Hepatitis A and E are transmitted by the faecal–oral route and are frequently acquired in countries where sanitation is poor (e.g. in Asia and Africa). Hepatitis B is transmitted parenterally and has a high prevalence in areas such as Asia and Africa. Sexual contact or surgery or receipt of blood products in such a country should be enquired about.

• *Is there any family history?* There is a genetic component to some of the prehepatic causes of jaundice. For example, glucose-6-phosphate dehydrogenase (G6PD) deficiency is an X-linked recessive condition and haemolysis can be precipitated by antimalarial medication.

• *Has he been in contact with anyone with a similar illness?* Infection with hepatitis A and occasionally hepatitis E can result in outbreaks in communities.

• *Does he have any risk factors for transmissible hepatitis?* A sexual history should be obtained as well as a history of intravenous drug use. Enquiries should be made about receipt of blood products, surgery in underdeveloped countries, tattoos and body piercing. As some hepatitis viruses can have incubation periods of as long as 6 months it is important to extend the history taking over that period.

• *What is his alcohol intake?* Alcohol is a common cause of jaundice and should always be specifically enquired about.

• *Has he taken any medication?* Prescribed and recreational drugs should be asked about. Antibiotics and herbal remedies are often taken and forgotten about so

Hepatology: Clinical Cases Uncovered, 1st edition. © Kathryn Nash and Indra Neil Guha. Published 2011 by Blackwell Publishing Ltd.

specifically ask about these. Drugs can cause a hepatocellular or cholestatic hepatitis.

Mr Farrelly describes no change in colour of his stools or urine. His abdominal discomfort is mild and left sided but is constant. There has been no recent travel abroad, he denies any recreational drugs or recent medications and he is teetotal. He is unaware of any family history of jaundice.

What clinical signs would you look for?

In addition to excluding signs of chronic liver disease the following may be useful to look for in this case:

• Confirm the presence of jaundice by examining the sclera.
• Hepatosplenomegaly and lymphadenopathy may imply an underlying haematological disorder.
• Tenderness in the right upper quadrant may suggest gallstones.
• Kayser–Fleischer rings in the eyes are associated with Wilson's disease.

On examination Mr Farrelly is jaundiced. He has mild splenomegaly and axillary lymphadenopathy. No signs of chronic liver disease are seen. Blood tests reveal the following:

Bilirubin	*48 μmol/L*
ALT	*28 iU/L*
ALP	*95 iU/L*
Albumin	*36 g/L*
Hb	*13.6 g/dL*
WBC	*6.7 × 10⁹/L*
Plt	*520 × 10⁹/L*

What additional investigations would be helpful?

The liver function tests are all normal except for an isolated hyperbilirubinaemia. This is suggestive of a prehepatic jaundice. The major differential diagnosis is an overproduction of bilirubin (e.g. haemolysis) or disturbance of bilirubin conjugation. The following investigations would be helpful:

• *Conjugated/unconjugated bilirubin*: An elevated unconjugated bilirubin (indirect) would confirm a prehepatic cause of jaundice. In the absence of haemolysis this would suggest an inherited disorder of conjugation such as Gilbert's syndrome or Crigler–Najjar syndrome.
• *Haemolysis screen*: This includes a blood film for fragmented red blood cells; an absolute reticulocyte count;

plasma levels of haptoglobin; and haemosiderin detection in the urine.
• *Viral serology*: The absence of a transaminitis suggests that this is not a viral hepatitis. The splenomegaly and lymphadenopathy imply this, however, could be due to a systemic viral infection and serology for Epstein–Barr virus (EBV) and cytomegalovirus (CMV) would be useful.

Further investigations show an indirect bilirubin of 35 μmol/L and a direct bilirubin of 13 μmol/L. The haemolysis screen is negative. Serology shows the presence of high EBV IgM titres suggestive of recent infection. The likely diagnosis is therefore that of Gilbert's syndrome (Box 1.1) with jaundice precipitated by an intercurrent illness (EBV infection).

Box 1.1 Gilbert's syndrome

• Prevalence is approximately 5% in Western society
• It results from a genetic defect in UGT1A1 on chromosome 2 (autosomal recessive) and results in decreased hepatic glucuronidation (by approximately 30%)
• Fasting will increase bilirubin levels and this can be a useful diagnostic test
• Bilirubin levels are usually less than 100 μmol/L
• Liver biopsy is not necessary and if performed is normal
• The condition is entirely benign and associated with a normal lifespan
• It is a related condition of the Crigler–Najjar syndrome. Type 1 results in a complete absence of conjugating enzyme with severe hyperbilirubinaemia, usually presenting in early life. In type 2, the conjugating enzyme is reduced to less than 10%. The bilirubinaemia in type 2 is usually higher than Gilbert's syndrome but molecular analysis can distinguish these two conditions

---

What treatment and further follow-up would you recommend?

The jaundice will improve and no specific treatment is required. Reassurance should be given to the patient. It is also important to warn them that future episodes may occur and be precipitated by illness or fasting. Regular follow-up in a liver clinic is not required. It would be extremely rare for EBV to produce a chronic hepatitis although not uncommon for it to be associated with a prolonged period of fatigue.

CASE REVIEW

A young man presented with jaundice and isolated elevation in bilirubin. The absence of derangement in other liver function tests and raised indirect bilirubin levels was suggestive of a disorder in conjugation or haemolysis.

The negative haemolysis screen was helpful in establishing the diagnosis of Gilbert's syndrome precipitated by an intercurrent illness (acute EBV infection).

KEY POINTS

- An isolated hyperbilirubinaemia in the absence of a transaminitis suggests a prehepatic cause for the jaundice
- A haemolysis screen and separation of bilirubin into 'direct' and 'indirect' components are important tests for prehepatic jaundice
- The management of Gilbert's syndrome is conservative
- The long-term prognosis of Gilbert's syndrome is excellent; patients have a normal lifespan and require no active intervention

Case 2 A 25-year-old man with nausea, vomiting and jaundice

Brian Dixon is a 25-year-old chemical engineer who presents to his general practitioner with generalised symptoms of malaise, anorexia and fever. He is normally fit and well but began to feel ill 2 weeks after returning from a holiday to rural India. During the consultation the GP notices that he is jaundiced.

What questions would you ask him?
• How long has he had these symptoms?
• Has he had a similar illness before?
• Is there a history of pain?
• Have there been any changes to the colour of the urine or stool?
• Has there been any weight loss?
• Is there a family history of liver disease or similar illnesses?
• Has he been in contact with anyone with a similar illness?
• Does he have any risk factors for transmissible hepatitis?
• What is his country of origin?
• What is his past medical history?
• Has he taken any medication or other substance?
A more detailed account of the history required in a patient presenting with jaundice is given in Case 1.

What signs would you look for on examination?
The history is suggestive of an episode of viral hepatitis and findings such as lymphadenopathy and hepatosplenomegaly are to be expected. It is also important to exclude more serious presentations that might require urgent attention in hospital. Your examination therefore needs to address two important questions:

1 *Are there signs of liver failure?* In acute liver injury the most important fact to ascertain is whether the liver is functioning. It is very rare for an acute liver injury to result in liver failure, but if it does occur it does so very quickly and there is only a very narrow window to intervene to save the patient's life. Signs of encephalopathy should be sought for such as impaired concentration or confusion, and the presence of a hepatic asterixis should be looked for.

2 *Are there signs of chronic liver disease?* Signs of chronic liver disease such as palmar erythema, spider naevi and splenomegaly should be sought as their presence is more suggestive of a longstanding process. Their absence, however, does not exclude a chronic liver disease.

On examination Mr Dixon does not have any signs of chronic liver disease, there is no hepatic fetor or asterixis and his cognition appears normal. In his abdomen his liver is palpable 2 cm below the costal margin but there is no splenomegaly or ascites. His blood test results come back later that day:

Bilirubin	*87 µmol/L*
ALT	*1842 iU/L*
ALP	*176 iU/L*
Albumin	*38 g/L*
CRP	*5 mg/L*

What does this pattern of blood tests suggest?
The striking elevation in ALT suggests inflammation of the parenchyma of the liver, which is known as hepatitis. ALT is present intracellularly in hepatocytes and is released into the blood in response to hepatocyte injury and necrosis. The C-reactive protein (CRP) is normal making a bacterial infection unlikely.

Hepatology: Clinical Cases Uncovered, 1st edition. © Kathryn Nash and Indra Neil Guha. Published 2011 by Blackwell Publishing Ltd.

What are the differential diagnoses for acute hepatitis?

• *Acute viral hepatitis*: In a young, previously well person, acute viral hepatitis is the most likely diagnosis. This may be caused by a directly hepatotrophic virus or by another virus that causes hepatitis as part of a multi-system illness (e.g. CMV, EBV).

• *Acute autoimmune hepatitis*: This is a rare cause of jaundice but it is important as it needs urgent referral to hospital for diagnosis and treatment to limit the degree of liver damage.

• *Drug-related liver injury*: A variety of drugs may cause liver injury. Diagnosis is important to prevent ongoing damage and to ensure that the drug is avoided in the future.

• *Metabolic cause*: Rare metabolic disorders that can present acutely should always be considered, particularly in young people (e.g. Wilson's disease).

• *Others*: A variety of other processes can cause acute liver injury and should be considered, e.g. vascular disorders (ischaemic hepatitis, venous thrombosis), lymphoma and pregnancy. Other rare causes include mushroom poisoning and injury related to toxins or chemicals. In a significant number of cases no cause is identified and the illness is called seronegative hepatitis.

What other important blood test should be done?

The single most important test is one to assess the synthetic function of the liver. This is best achieved by testing blood coagulation with either a prothrombin time (PT) or international normalised ratio (INR) since most of the factors required for blood clotting are synthesised within the liver. Impairment of this process is a marker of severe liver injury and any patient with a suspected acute liver injury and impaired coagulation must be immediately referred to hospital.

The traditional 'liver function tests' (bilirubin, transaminases and alkaline phosphatase) do not actually test liver function and are unhelpful when determining if there is liver failure requiring urgent referral to hospital. Elevation in these blood tests is variable and of no prognostic value. For example, in acute viral hepatitis, hepatic necrosis commonly results in an ALT of several thousand but a normal INR. This indicates that there is liver cell damage but that adequate synthetic function remains.

KEY POINT

• In an acute liver injury the most important test is to make an assessment of blood clotting with either prothrombin time or INR. The result must be obtained that day and if there is impairment of coagulation the patient must be referred to hospital immediately

---

What further tests would you organise?

• *Acute viral hepatitis screen*: In acute illness it is important to look for evidence of recent viral infection and to differentiate this from past exposure, vaccination or chronic infection. IgM antibodies are the first antibodies produced in response to infection and, therefore, the presence of IgM antibodies to viruses known to cause acute hepatitis should be sought (Table 2.1).

• *Autoimmune screen*: An immunological assessment is required including immunoglobulins, antinuclear antibody (ANA) and liver-specific antibodies (anti smooth muscle antibody, anti-liver/kidney microsomal antibody, antimitochondrial antibody).

• *Metabolic screen*: Blood should be sent to test for caeruloplasmin and copper to investigate the possibility of Wilson's disease.

• *Urea and electrolytes*: Severe liver injury can occasionally cause renal failure. Electrolyte disturbance is common especially if there is nausea and anorexia leading to poor

Table 2.1 Viral serological testing in suspected acute liver injury.

Virus	Antibody response
Hepatitis A virus	Anti-HAV IgM antibody
Hepatitis B virus	Hepatitis B anti-core IgM antibody (HBcAb)*
Hepatitis C virus	Anti-HCV antibody[†]
Hepatitis E virus	Anti-HEV IgM antibody
Cytomegalovirus	Anti-CMV IgM antibody
Epstein–Barr virus	Anti-EBV IgM antibody
Herpes simplex virus	Anti-HSV IgM antibody

* Several antibodies are produced in response to hepatitis B infection. IgM anti-core antibody is the best test for recent infection.

[†] Hepatitis C antibody testing is an IgG antibody test. If this infection is suspected and the test is negative it should be repeated 3 months later.

Table 2.2 Features of some hepatitis viruses that cause acute hepatitis.

	Hepatitis A	Hepatitis B	Hepatitis C	Hepatitis D	Hepatitis E
Virus	RNA Picornavirus	DNA Hepadnavirus	RNA Flavivirus	RNA Subviral particle	RNA Calcivirus
Spread	Faecal–oral	Blood Sexual Vertical	Blood Sexual (rare) Vertical (rare)	Blood Sexual	Faecal–oral
Incubation period	Short 2–4 weeks	Long 2–6 months	Intermediate 4–12 weeks	Intermediate 4–8 weeks	Short 2–8 weeks
Acute infection	Yes	Yes	Yes, but rarely symptomatic	Yes	Yes
Mortality (acute)	<0.5%	<1%	<1%		1–2% (pregnant women 10–20%)
Carrier state	No	Yes	Yes	Yes	No
Chronic infection	No	Yes	Yes	Yes	No
Vaccine	Yes	Yes	No	No, but can be prevented by HBV vaccination	No

oral intake or there is a history of diarrhoea and vomiting.

• *Full blood count*: An eosinophilia may suggest a drug-induced liver injury.

• *Liver imaging*: Ultrasound is the most helpful screening test. It is necessary to exclude biliary obstruction, to look for signs of chronic liver disease (splenomegaly, varices, portal hypertension) and to assess patency of hepatic vessels.

What viruses can cause acute hepatitis?

• Hepatitis A
• Hepatitis B
• Hepatitis E
• Hepatitis C (this is a rare cause of acute hepatitis, infection is usually asymptomatic)
• Hepatitis D (either co-infection with hepatitis B or superadded infection of someone chronically infected with hepatitis B)
• Cytomegalovirus (CMV)
• Epstein–Barr virus (EBV)
• Herpes simplex virus (HSV)
• Yellow fever (Table 2.2).

Mr Dixon's INR is normal; 5 days later the results of further blood tests are available:

Hepatitis A	*IgM negative, IgG positive*
Hepatitis B	*HBsAg negative, anti-core IgM negative*
Hepatitis C	*Anti-HCV negative*
Hepatitis E	*IgM positive, IgG negative*
CMV	*IgM negative, IgG negative*
EBV	*IgM negative, IgG positive*
HSV	*IgM negative, IgG negative*

What is the diagnosis?

Acute hepatitis E infection.

How do you interpret the viral serology?

• He has a positive IgM antibody against hepatitis E virus and has not yet produced an IgG antibody, indicating recent infection.

• The absence of hepatitis A IgM antibody excludes acute hepatitis A infection. He has a positive IgG antibody against this virus, which could have occurred due to previous infection or vaccination. Prior to travelling to an endemic area such as India, vaccination is strongly recommended.

• He has evidence of previous exposure to EBV (glandular fever) but not acute infection.

• There is no evidence of past or current infection with hepatitis B, hepatitis C, CMV or HSV.

How should the patient be managed?

Treatment of acute viral hepatitis is symptomatic and the majority of patients recover completely. Most cases can be managed at home unless there is a suggestion that the patient has or may develop liver failure (derangement of coagulation, encephalopathy). This patient has markedly deranged liver function tests suggesting a severe liver injury but he does not have evidence of coagulopathy at this point. Given that he is jaundiced, he should have daily blood tests until it is clear that he is not developing a coagulopathy and the liver function tests are starting to improve. Provided that these tests can be taken and reviewed promptly he can be managed in the community.

What else must you do?

Cases of viral hepatitis should be notified to the Health Protection Agency who will investigate the potential source. This is an important public health measure to try to limit future outbreaks.

Mr Dixon is seen daily by his GP and his bloods improve. Six weeks later he feels fully recovered and his liver function tests have returned to normal. Convalescent serology reveals a positive IgG antibody against hepatitis E and the IgM antibody is no longer detectable.

CASE REVIEW

This man is normally fit and healthy but presented with an acute illness characterised by non-specific symptoms of nausea and anorexia. He was jaundiced and blood tests revealed a significantly elevated ALT consistent with hepatic inflammation and necrosis. On examination there were no signs of encephalopathy or chronic liver disease. His INR was normal suggesting that the liver was still capable of synthetic function. Further blood tests revealed that he had acute infection with hepatitis E virus. His jaundice settled and he made a full recovery. Convalescent serology was in keeping with a recent acute hepatitis E infection as evidenced by the loss of IgM antibody and the development of IgG antibody.

KEY POINTS

• Acute viral hepatitis is a common cause of liver injury. It is usually self-limiting and patients make a full recovery

• It is rare for patients with acute viral hepatitis to develop liver failure but if it does occur it does so very rapidly. Therefore any patient presenting with jaundice needs to be carefully evaluated to ensure that they are not going to develop liver failure

• The most important test of liver function is a test of the liver's ability to synthesise proteins of the coagulation cascade. This is provided by either the prothrombin time or INR. If there is evidence of coagulopathy then the patient should be admitted to hospital that day

• Patients presenting with acute liver injury should be asked a thorough history to try to elicit important risk factors

• Most patients with viral hepatitis can be managed in the community with symptomatic treatment

A 45-year-old woman presenting with severe right upper quadrant pain and jaundice

Mrs Emma Watson is a 45-year-old artist who presents with a 2-day history of right upper quadrant pain and jaundice. She has noticed her stools are light and her urine is a darker colour than usual. She has been seen in the emergency department and you have been asked to review her. On examination she is apyrexial, in pain and distressed. Her blood pressure is 130/80 mmHg and pulse is 80 beats per minute. She has mild tenderness in the right upper quadrant but no rebound or guarding. Blood tests have returned and show the following:

Bilirubin	*79 μmol/L*
ALT	*67 iU/L*
ALP	*587 iU/L*
Albumin	*39 g/L*
γ-GT	*784 U/L*

What pattern of abnormality is seen in her blood tests?

She is jaundiced as evidenced by a raised bilirubin. The alkaline phosphatase and γ-GT are elevated suggesting that the problem is biliary in nature (i.e. a cholestatic jaundice). This may occur due to extrahepatic or intrahepatic biliary disease although her history of pain is suggestive of an extrahepatic cause.

What diagnoses would you wish to consider at this stage?

The important diagnoses to consider are:

• *Posthepatic jaundice from gallstones*: A gallstone can cause an obstructive picture if it becomes lodged anywhere from the gallbladder to the ampulla of Vater (Fig. 3.1).

• *Cholecystitis*: Inflammation of the gallbladder can present acutely with pain and derangement of liver function tests (Box 3.1).

• *Gallstone pancreatitis*: Acute pancreatitis can be precipitated by gallstones becoming lodged in the common bile duct and is an indication for urgent endoscopic intervention.

• *Perforated viscus*: The other differentials for severe abdominal pain should be excluded, e.g. a perforated peptic ulcer, appendicitis, kidney stones, etc. Rarely, a gallstone can erode through the biliary tract and present as a perforation. If the gallstone reaches the small bowel it can cause obstruction or gallstone ileus (Fig. 3.2).

• *Chronic biliary obstruction*: If the history was over a longer period of time other causes of obstruction (e.g. stricture to the common bile duct, cholangiocarcinoma and a tumour in the head of the pancreas) should be considered. Sometimes these cases present acutely when an asymptomatic chronic obstruction reaches a critical aperture of bile duct narrowing.

What are the next steps in management of this woman?

• *Ensure adequate resuscitation*: As with the management of any acutely unwell patient the first step is to check that her airway, breathing and circulation are not compromised. Establishing early intravenous access is a prudent measure in this scenario in view of the early differential diagnoses.

• *Analgesia*: Treating her pain is an important early intervention and intravenous analgesia may be the most effective way of dealing with this quickly. Opiates can theoretically increase biliary pressure and spasm and often non-steroidal anti-inflammatory drugs (NSAIDs) in combination with antispasmodics are used to relieve pain.

• *Further investigations*:
  ○ Amylase: to exclude pancreatitis.

Hepatology: Clinical Cases Uncovered, 1st edition. © Kathryn Nash and Indra Neil Guha. Published 2011 by Blackwell Publishing Ltd.

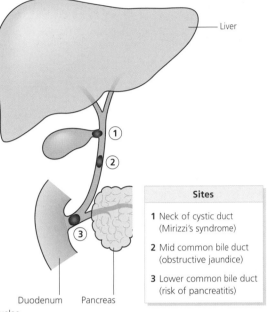

Figure 3.1 Gallstones and clinical sequelae.

Liver

Duodenum   Pancreas

Sites
1 Neck of cystic duct (Mirizzi's syndrome)
2 Mid common bile duct (obstructive jaundice)
3 Lower common bile duct (risk of pancreatitis)

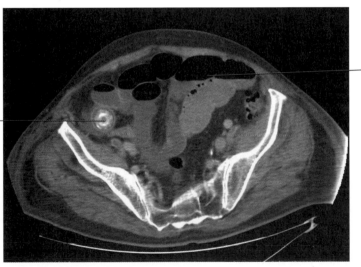

Gallstone within bowel lumen

Dilated bowel loops

Figure 3.2 Gallstone ileus.

Box 3.1 Features of cholecystitis

- Pain: the classic description of biliary colic is of pain radiating around like a band from the back. Pain may be elicited on palpation in the right upper quadrant (Murphy's sign)
- Sepsis: pyrexia, raised white cell count or C-reactive protein
- Deranged liver function tests: an inflamed gallbladder often does not cause jaundice as it does not impair bile flow. If a gallstone becomes lodged in the cystic duct, however, this can impair bile flow in the common bile duct and result in jaundice (Mirizzi's syndrome (see Fig. 3.1))
- Gallstones are the commonest cause of cholecystitis but it can occur in their absence (acalculous cholecystitis) as a result of ischaemia

○ Erect chest X-ray (CXR): the presence of subdiaphragmatic air should alert you to the possibility of perforation.

○ An urgent ultrasound scan: this will give information on whether the biliary system is dilated or not. Ultrasound may miss the presence of stones in the common bile duct but the presence of intrahepatic duct dilatation in the context of this case would strongly suggest biliary obstruction.

What further investigations can be helpful in the assessment of patients with obstructive jaundice?

• Magnetic resonance cholangiopancreatography (MRCP) can give better resolution of the biliary tree than ultrasound. It is a safer modality than endoscopic retrograde cholangiopancreatography (ERCP) for the diagnosis of gallstones.

• Endoscopic ultrasound (EUS) can be useful in diagnostic uncertainty to detect gallstones in the common bile duct.

Mrs Watson's amylase is normal and an erect CXR does not show any evidence of free air. An urgent ultrasound is arranged and shows dilated intrahepatic bile ducts (Fig. 3.3) and a filling defect in the mid common bile duct suggestive of a large gallstone. On arrival back on the ward you are

urgently called. Her blood pressure is 90/60mmHg with a pulse rate of 100 beats per minute and her temperature is 38.5°C.

What is the most likely cause of her deterioration?

The most likely cause is ascending cholangitis. She has evidence of Charcot's triad (fever, jaundice and right upper quadrant pain) which is characteristic of this very serious condition.

How would you mange her now?
Resuscitation

She is showing signs of shock. She needs resuscitation using the basic principle of airway, breathing and circulation:

• High dose oxygen.

• Ensure adequate intravenous access and commence intravenous fluids.

• Insert a urinary catheter to monitor urinary output.

• Monitor the response to bolus intravenous fluids. Consider the need for invasive monitoring of her central blood volume (CVP lines) if the blood pressure and pulse do not respond.

• Consider where the best environment is for her to be managed; consider transfer to a high dependency unit.

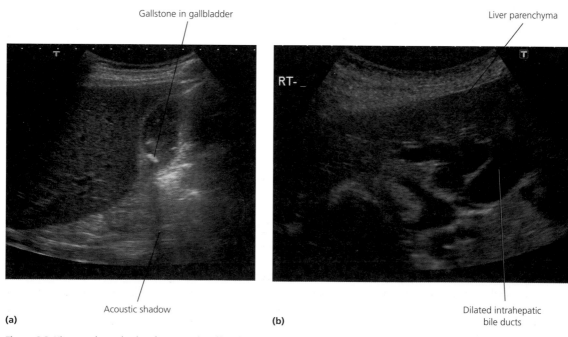

Gallstone in gallbladder

Liver parenchyma

RT-

Acoustic shadow

Dilated intrahepatic bile ducts

(a) **(b)**

Figure 3.3 Ultrasound examination demonstrating dilated intrahepatic bile ducts.

Table 3.1 Examples of organisms seen in ascending cholangitis.

Organism	Therapy options
Gram negative, e.g. *Escherichia coli*, *Klebsiella*, *Enterobacter* spp	Clavulanic acid + amoxicillin Piperacillin Cefuroxime Cefotaxime Ciprofloxacin Imipenem/meropenem
Anaerobes, e.g. *Bacteroides* spp, *Clostridium* spp	Metronidazole Imipenem/meropenem
Anaerobes, e.g. *Pseudomonas*	Piperacillin Ciprofloxacin Imipenem/meropenem

Antibiotic therapy

Blood cultures are taken to identify the organism responsible for her infection and to determine sensitivities to antibiotics. Broad spectrum antibiotics should be commenced. The likely organisms that cause infection in the biliary tree are shown in Table 3.1. It is important to use an antibiotic that will cover Gram-negative organisms.

> Mrs Watson responds to intravenous fluid therapy. Her blood pressure is now 120/80 mmHg and pulse 70 beats per minute. She has a good urine output. Blood cultures have been sent and antibiotic therapy with intravenous cephalosporin and metronidazole commenced. You are asked to look at some blood tests which were sent when she deteriorated:
>
> | | |
> |---|---|
> | Bilirubin | 160 μmol/L |
> | ALT | 187 iU/L |
> | ALP | 798 iU/L |
> | Albumin | 36 g/L |
> | γ-GT | 784 U/L |
> | Hb | 14.8 g/dL |
> | WBC | 14.4 × 10^9/L (neutrophilia) |
> | Plt | 478 × 10^9/L |

How should she be managed now?

Sepsis can cause a further deterioration in liver function tests *per se*. However, her obstructive picture has worsened. The major concern here is that she has an obstructed biliary system which is now infected. Without prompt drainage she may deteriorate further. ERCP could alleviate the obstruction (Box 3.2).

Box 3.2 ERCP procedure for common bile duct stones

- The patient is sedated and the endoscopist inserts a side viewing endoscope into the duodenum
- A cannula is inserted through the sphincter of Oddi into the common bile duct
- Contrast is injected, outlining the biliary tree (Fig. 3.4)
- A small cut can be made in the sphincter of Oddi using diathermy (sphincterotomy) which will ease the passage of gallstones into the duodenum (Fig. 3.5)
- A variety of techniques are available for the endoscopist to remove stones from the bile duct including crushing stones, retrieving them with baskets and inflating a balloon within the bile duct to literally pull them out
- If a bile duct stone cannot be removed endoscopically a stent can be inserted to bypass the blockage and allow bile to flow into the duodenum

> Mrs Watson has an urgent ERCP performed. This confirms the presence of a gallstone (Box 3.3) in the common bile duct (Fig. 3.4). A sphincterotomy is performed and the gallstone is removed (Fig. 3.5). Over the next few days her liver function tests improve.

What is the long-term plan?

Although Mrs Watson has had a sphincterotomy and had drainage she will need a definitive procedure to remove her gallbladder. She undergoes an elective laparoscopic cholecystectomy a few months later.

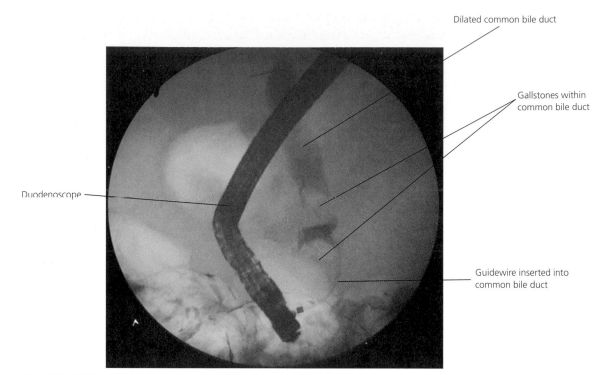

Dilated common bile duct

Gallstones within
common bile duct

Duodenoscope

Guidewire inserted into
common bile duct

Figure 3.4 ERCP examination demonstrating multiple gallstones in the common bile duct.

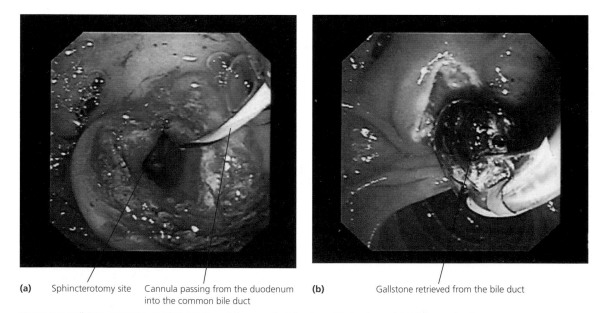

(a)   Sphincterotomy site   Cannula passing from the duodenum   **(b)**   Gallstone retrieved from the bile duct
into the common bile duct

Figure 3.5 Gallstone extraction at ERCP. (a) View of the ampulla following sphincterotomy. (b) Gallstone extraction.

Box 3.3 Gallstones

- The prevalence of gallstones is between 10% and 20% in Western societies. The vast majority of patients with chronic gallstones (60–80%) are asymptomatic
- Approximately 80% are cholesterol stones, the remainder being either pigment or mixed stones
- Cholesterol stones occur in patients who have an increase in the ratio of cholesterol : bile salts in the bile. Risk factors include:
  ○ increased age
  ○ obesity and high animal fat diet
  ○ hormonal: female sex, multiparity, contraceptive pill use
  ○ ileal disease or resection
  ○ diabetes
- Pigment stones contain an excess of bile pigments from excessive red cell breakdown, e.g. haemolytic anaemia
- Clinical presentation when it occurs may be as follows:
  ○ biliary pain or colic (intermittent obstruction of the cystic duct by a gallstone)
  ○ acute or chronic cholecystitis: this is precipitated by a gallstone or sludge in the cystic duct (the combination of raised intraluminal pressure and bile initiates an inflammatory reaction in the gallbladder wall)
  ○ jaundice: usually occurs as a result of a gallstone in the common bile duct but can occur if gallstones becoming

lodged in the neck of the cystic duct and the inflammatory mass then obstruct the common bile duct (Mirizzi's syndrome (see Fig. 3.1)
  ○ cholangitis
  ○ pancreatitis
  ○ fistulating disease: gallstones can erode through the biliary wall and cause subsequent obstruction of the duodenum (Bouveret's syndrome) or small bowel (gallstone ileus)
- The non-invasive diagnostic modalities for the detection of gallstones include ultrasound (may miss stones in the common bile duct), MRCP and EUS
- The standard treatment of chronic cholelithiasis is laparoscopic cholecystectomy
- Non-surgical techniques such as ursodeoxycholic acid and extracorporeal shockwave lithotripsy are associated with high rates of recurrence. In some centres these options are considered in selected patients (factors such as the size of the stones and constituency of the stones will determine success)
- In patients with stones in the common bile duct the options include a therapeutic ERCP with sphincterotomy or intraoperative bile duct exploration

CASE REVIEW

A 45-year-old woman presented with right upper quadrant pain with symptoms, signs and liver function tests suggesting an obstructive jaundice. Radiology revealed dilated intrahepatic ducts and a filling defect in the common bile duct. She developed sepsis with circulatory compromise and was resuscitated. Treatment was initiated with broad spectrum intravenous antibiotics. An urgent ERCP was performed and this relieved the obstruction with resolution of her symptoms and liver function tests.

KEY POINTS

- The presence of right upper quadrant pain associated with jaundice is highly suggestive of gallstones. Other causes of obstruction along the extrahepatic biliary tree need to be excluded
- Imaging of the biliary tree is vital to provide a prompt and accurate diagnosis
- Imaging modalities will range from easily accessible ultrasound to specialised tests such as MRCP or endoscopic ultrasound

- An obstructed biliary system is prone to biliary stasis and the risk of infection
- Ascending cholangitis is a medical emergency and requires prompt resuscitation and antibiotic therapy
- Ascending cholangitis is an urgent indication for ERCP to alleviate the obstruction and therefore treat the sepsis
- Long-term treatment for gallstones is cholecystectomy, which is usually performed by laparoscopy

Case 4 A 72-year-old man with painless jaundice

Mr Parakesh Rana is a 72-year-old man who presents to his GP with a 3-week history of painless jaundice. The GP asks him some relevant questions.

In addition to a comprehensive history what specific questions would you ask?
- Duration.
- Colour of stools and urine.
- Detailed drug history:
  ○ Medication
  ○ Herbal
  ○ Antibiotics
  ○ Recreational.
- Presence of constitutional symptoms: weight loss, pruritus and night sweats.
- Previous abdominal surgery.
- History of pancreatitis.
- Associated autoimmune phenomenon (e.g. vitiligo, pernicious anaemia, etc.).
- Detailed alcohol history.
- Potential indicators of pancreatic pathology:
  ○ Symptoms of diabetes or recent diagnosis of diabetes
  ○ Steatorrhoea.
- Gastric outflow obstruction.

Mr Rana has been previously well and has never been admitted to hospital before. His jaundice has become progressively more pronounced over 3 weeks and he describes a 12.5 kg weight loss over 3 months with some associated mild epigastric discomfort. His stools are very pale in colour, almost white, and his urine is dark. His only past medical history is psoriasis and there is no history of abdominal surgery. He admits to drinking approximately 30–40 units of alcohol per week, consisting of whisky at the weekends, since his early twenties. The GP has organised

Hepatology: Clinical Cases Uncovered, 1st edition. © Kathryn Nash and Indra Neil Guha. Published 2011 by Blackwell Publishing Ltd.

some liver function tests and an urgent ultrasound. The results of the investigations are:

Bilirubin	95 μmol/L
ALT	54 iU/L
ALP	787 iU/L
Albumin	28 g/L
Fasting blood glucose	8.9 mmol/L

Liver ultrasound: markedly dilated intrahepatic ducts with dilatation of the common bile duct. The lower common bile duct and pancreas cannot be adequately visualised. No gallstones are seen in the gallbladder. The spleen and kidneys are of normal size and appearance.

What are the differential diagnoses?
The major differentials include:
- Pancreatic carcinoma (Box 4.1).
- Chronic pancreatitis (Box 4.2).
- Autoimmune pancreatitis (Box 4.3).
- Extrapancreatic malignancy including cholangiocarcinoma, ampullary cancer, lymphoma, metastatic cancer or neuroendocrine tumour (Box 4.4).

What is the most appropriate investigation to consider next?
Cross-sectional imaging with a CT scan will help locate the level of the obstruction and may identify the cause. If the cause is malignant it may also indicate whether there is local, regional or more extensive involvement, which will guide future management.

An urgent CT scan is ordered and this reveals a pancreatic tumour with evidence of intrahepatic bile duct dilatation and gallbladder distension (Fig. 4.1). There is evidence of spread to local lymph nodes.

What investigation is needed next?
It is important to obtain a histological diagnosis to confirm the suspicion of pancreatic carcinoma. Several

Box 4.1 Pancreatic carcinoma

- Risk factors include smoking, diabetes, diet, previous partial gastrectomy and possibly alcohol consumption
- Males are affected more commonly than females and the majority of cases occur in patients over 50 years
- Classically, pancreatic cancer is described as painless progressive jaundice. In fact it can be associated with upper abdominal pain or back pain. Due to anatomical location of tumours of the head of the pancreas, they will present with symptoms of jaundice earlier than tumours arising in the body or tail
- A palpable gallbladder in the presence of jaundice is unlikely to be due to gallstones (Courvoisier's law) and it should alert the clinician to the possibility of a pancreatic tumour
- There are currently no specific blood tests for pancreatic cancer. Investigations may confirm jaundice, exocrine and endocrine insufficiency

Box 4.2 Chronic pancreatitis

- Alcohol is the commonest cause of chronic pancreatitis
- There may be associated strictures of the common bile duct or pancreatic ducts. The latter may result in tortuous and irregular pancreatic ducts with associated calcification
- Acute or chronic inflammation leading to pancreatic necrosis can result in the formation of pancreatic pseudocysts. These can cause obstruction leading to abdominal discomfort or impedence of biliary and pancreatic drainage

Box 4.3 Autoimmune pancreatitis

- This is a relatively new concept characterised by an inflammatory process, with the presence of IgG4 subtype plasma cells
- It is an important diagnosis to consider as it may mimic clinical features of pancreatic malignancy or benign strictures in the biliary tree and will respond to immunosuppression
- The patient may exhibit other features of autoimmune phenomena (Sjögren's syndrome, vitiligo, pernicious anaemia, etc.)

methods are available for obtaining pancreatic tissue (Box 4.5).

An endoscopic ultrasound confirms a mass within the head of the pancreas with lymphadenopathy. The mass is seen to be invading the superior mesenteric vein. A biopsy taken during the procedure demonstrates adenocarcinoma.

Box 4.4 Extrapancreatic malignancy

- Obstruction from the confluence of the left and right hepatic bile ducts to the ampulla of Vater may lead to obstructive jaundice, for example:
  - intrahepatic and porta hepatitis: lymphoma, metastatic carcinoma, neuroendocrine tumour
  - common bile duct: cholangiocarcinoma
  - gallbladder cancer
- The prognosis may be very different; for example lymphoma with hepatic dissemination can still have a 5-year survival of 85%, and ampullary cancer, if limited to the duodenal mucosa, has reported survival rates of 90%
- Histological confirmation is therefore not simply academic and can alter management

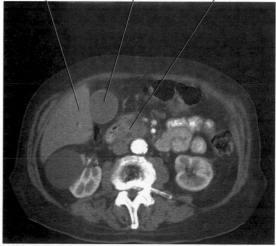

Dilated intrahepatic ducts | Distended gallbladder | Mass in the head of the pancreas

Figure 4.1 CT scan demonstrating biliary obstruction caused by a pancreatic tumour.

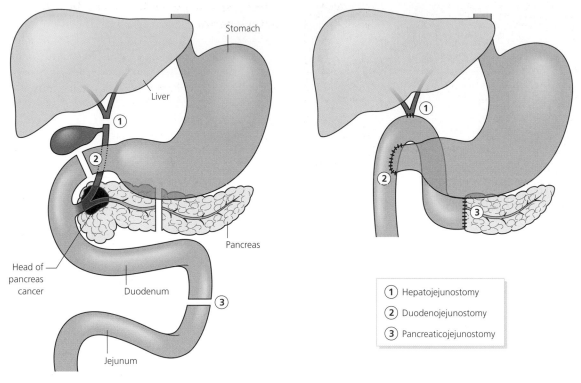

(a) Before, demonstrating sites of resection

(b) After, demonstrating the three anastomoses

Figure 4.2 Whipple's procedure. (a) Before demonstrating sites of resection. (b) After demonstrating the three anastomoses.

> **Box 4.5 Techniques for obtaining pancreatic histology**
>
> - Endoscopic ultrasound with fine needle aspiration or trucut biopsy
> - CT or ultrasound-guided percutaneous biopsy
> - Biopsy under direct vision at surgery

What are the possible management approaches for pancreatic carcinoma?

Surgery

- Surgical resection will depend on the extent of the tumour and specifically if there has been invasion into the major vessels including the superior mesenteric vein and portal vein, evidence of metastatic spread and suitability of the patient for major abdominal surgery.
- Whipple's procedure, when performed in appropriate centres, carries a perioperative mortality of 0–3% and the

5-year survival is between 20% and 40%. Figure 4.2 is a simplified diagram of the procedure. It should be noted that only 20% of patients are eligible for curative resection and the overall survival for pancreatic cancer at 5 years remains approximately 5%.

Chemotherapy

- Systemic chemotherapy can be given. There is continuing research in this area but at the time of writing life expectancy has been shown to improve by between 2 to 7 months in those given chemotherapy in large clinical trials.
- Side effects of chemotherapy include nausea, bone marrow suppression and hair loss.
- Careful discussion with an experienced oncologist and patient is vital in deciding the risk:benefit ratio.

Stenting of the common bile duct (Fig. 4.3)

- This will relieve jaundice but does nothing for the underlying neoplastic process.

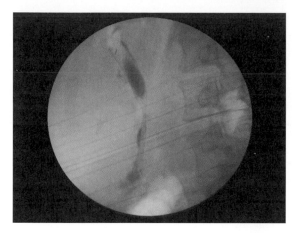

Figure 4.3 Radiograph demonstrating biliary stent inserted at ERCP.

• Stenting may be performed as a temporary measure to allow jaundice to settle prior to proceeding to surgery or it may be a purely palliative manoeuvre.

• The choice is between inserting a plastic stent and a metal stent:

○ A plastic stent is often considered if surgery is being contemplated as they are more easily removed during the operation (although novel metal stents that can be removed are available).

○ The stent occlusion rate is greater with plastic stents.

○ Metal stents are more expensive.

○ The choice of stents for palliation thus depends on the anticipated progression of the tumour. If the patient is expected to survive more than 3 months, a metal stent is usually inserted.

The tumour is deemed too extensive for surgical resection. An appointment is made with the oncologist. The advantages of chemotherapy, including the potential to prolong survival, and the disadvantages, including the side effects of chemotherapy, are discussed. Mr Rana opts not to have chemotherapy. An ERCP is organised and a metallic stent is inserted to relieve the jaundice.

Mr Rana goes home with his metal stent and his jaundice improves slowly over 7 days. He is commenced on insulin during his hospital stay and his blood sugars are well controlled with this regime. He is reviewed by the Macmillan nurse specialist and is commenced on some regular analgesia which controls his pain. Three months after returning home Mr Rana presents to his GP with severe vomiting.

What are the possible causes for his deterioration?

• *Duodenal obstruction*: Growth of pancreatic tumours may result in duodenal obstruction leading to gastric outflow obstruction. This can lead to early satiety and vomiting occurring shortly after meals. A duodenal stent can be inserted to relieve the obstruction or a palliative bypass surgery undertaken.

• *Side effects of medication or disease progression*: The cancer itself can be associated with worsening symptoms of nausea and vomiting. The common analgesics used to alleviate pain are also associated with side effects of nausea. Therefore, specialist advice from the palliative care team is very important for the right combination of medication but also for the holistic care of the patient, as outlined in Box 4.6.

Mr Rana is found to have duodenal obstruction and a duodenal stent is inserted by a combined endoscopic and radiological approach. His condition continues to deteriorate and he is admitted to a hospice. He dies 2 weeks later and is surrounded by his family at this time.

Box 4.6 Palliative care of patients with pancreatic cancer

Broad principles

• Take a holistic approach considering physical, psychological, social and spiritual aspects of care

• It is important to involve the GP, district nurses, Macmillan nurses and palliative care team for complicated cases or those requiring hospice care

• Communication and support should be provided to both the patient and the family, including:

○ breaking bad news

○ end of life care

○ support in bereavement

Symptom control

• Medication, e.g. analgesia, antiemetics, etc.

• Nerve block for pain, e.g. coeliac plexus nerve block

• Stent insertion to blocked bile ducts (using ERCP or PTC)

• Bypass surgery: to bypass a blocked bile duct to treat jaundice

• Palliative chemotherapy

CASE REVIEW

A 72-year-old man presented with painless, obstructive jaundice. He had a previous history of alcohol dependence. Investigations, including a CT scan and biopsy of the lesion, revealed pancreatic cancer. The obstructive jaundice was relieved by a metal stent inserted at ERCP. His pancreatic cancer grew further, causing duodenal obstruction. His symptoms of gastric outflow obstruction were alleviated by the insertion of a further metal stent into the duodenum. He was actively managed by the palliative care team and was admitted to a hospice before he died.

KEY POINTS

- The causes of painless jaundice include benign and malignant aetiologies
- The type of malignancy is important to determine as the treatment and prognosis may differ
- The suspicion of pancreatic cancer should be high in the context of painless jaundice, especially if there are associated symptoms of endocrine disturbance
- Whipple's procedure is a potentially curative treatment for pancreatic cancer but only a minority of patients are eligible for curative surgery
- In those unsuitable for surgical resection, placement of a metal stent, to alleviate jaundice, may be appropriate
- Pancreatic cancer can cause gastric outflow obstruction and this differential should be considered in patients presenting with vomiting or early satiety
- Involvement of the palliative care team early in advanced pancreatic cancer is important for both the patient and their families

Case 5 A 23-year-old woman with vomiting and epigastric pain

Miranda Smith is brought into the emergency department by her friend as she has been vomiting and complaining of epigastric pain. Her friend reports that she broke up with her boyfriend a month ago and she has become depressed and increasingly withdrawn. On examination she has bilateral subconjunctival haemorrhages and is jaundiced with tenderness on palpation of her abdomen. Liver function tests reveal:

Bilirubin	*157 µmol/L*
ALT	*6362 iU/L*
ALP	*220 iU/L*
Albumin	*32 g/L*

What is the most likely diagnosis?

The history of a relationship breakdown and subsequent depression suggests the possibility that she has attempted suicide. In a patient presenting with symptoms and signs of an acute liver injury in this setting, a paracetamol (acetaminophen) overdose is the most likely diagnosis. Paracetamol overdose is the commonest cause of acute liver failure in the United Kingdom and accounts for over half of cases.

What further questions should be asked?

• The patient should be asked about the possibility of an overdose. Collateral history from the friend should be sought, e.g. were there any empty bottles at home, was there a suicide note?

• *How many tablets were taken?* The common threshold for liver damage to occur from a single paracetamol overdose is 10 g (20 tablets) although patients can sometimes ingest much larger quantities without sustaining significant liver injury. Significant hepatotoxicity has been reported following overdose of much smaller amounts,

however, particularly if the patient is taking enzyme-inducing drugs such as antiepileptics or has chronic alcohol ingestion.

• *When did the overdose occur?* It is important to establish how long ago the overdose took place. This will aid understanding of the significance of paracetamol levels in the blood and also give an indication of the prognosis and likely benefit of the specific antedote. Furthermore, whether the overdose was taken all in one setting or whether it was staggered over several hours or days should be ascertained. In the latter case, irreversible liver damage may already have occurred and the algorithms commonly used to guide referral for specialist care and liver transplantation are unreliable.

• *Was anything else taken with the paracetamol tablets?* Mixed overdoses are common and can present a confusing picture. For example, non-steroidal anti-inflammatory drug (NSAID) overdose may also cause hepatic and renal damage and produce similar symptoms to a paracetamol overdose. The possibility of additional ingestion of benzodiazepines or opiates should always be considered, particularly as paracetamol may be prescribed in tablets that contain opiates in addition, such as co-codamol or co-dydramol. Overdose of these substances, particularly in combination with alcohol, can lead to respiratory depression which can be rapidly fatal. In a mixed overdose drowsiness may respond to a specific antidote with flumazenil (for benzodiazepines) or naloxone (for opiates). If the patient does not respond to these antidotes or has taken a pure paracetamol overdose, drowsiness is an ominous sign that may suggest encephalopathy and the patient should be immediately discussed with a liver transplant centre.

• *Is there any evidence of pre-existing liver disease?* Patients with pre-existing liver disease who develop a superadded acute liver injury may be affected more severely. They may be more likely to decompensate and develop liver failure. Furthermore, the prognostic markers for paracetamol overdose are not valid in this situation.

Hepatology: Clinical Cases Uncovered, 1st edition. © Kathryn Nash and Indra Neil Guha. Published 2011 by Blackwell Publishing Ltd.

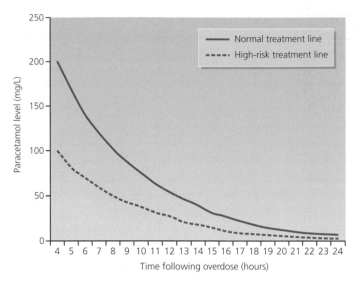

Figure 5.1 Nomogram for paracetamol dose taken, indicating when treatment should be given.

!RED FLAG

In some situations a patient with a paracetamol overdose may behave differently. Always consider the possibility of a mixed or staggered overdose. Both these situations may complicate the assessment of the patient and alter the value of prognostic criteria. *If in doubt always discuss the patient with a liver transplant unit.*

Miranda is reluctant to give a history but her friend reports that she hadn't seen her for 2 days. When she entered her flat there were empty bottles of paracetamol by the side of the bed.

What further investigations would you undertake?
Paracetamol level
Blood for paracetamol level should be taken if an overdose is suspected. In order to interpret the result it is essential to know accurately when the overdose took place:
- If the patient presents within 4 hours of overdose, the blood test should be delayed since serum levels drawn within 4 hours may not represent peak levels.
- The probability of hepatotoxicity can be ascertained using the graph in Fig. 5.1. The graph should only be used in relation to a single acute ingestion.
- A negative paracetamol level does not exclude a paracetamol overdose as liver failure occurs 72 hours after the

overdose at a time when paracetamol is no longer detectable in the blood.

!RED FLAG

A patient presenting with paracetamol-induced liver failure will usually have an undetectable level of paracetamol in the blood as the drug has already been metabolised. In the setting of acute liver failure, a negative paracetamol level does not exclude the diagnosis of paracetamol overdose.

Coagulation screen
All patients should have a coagulation screen performed to look specifically at the prothrombin time or international normalised ratio (INR). It is vital to ascertain whether the liver damage is causing impairment in its ability to synthesis proteins. The proteins of the coagulation cascade are synthesised in the liver and disturbance of this process occurs early in liver failure and may suggest that referral to a specialist centre is required.

Unless the patient is on warfarin or there is life-threatening bleeding it is important not to make any attempts to correct abnormalities in blood coagulation as this will invalidate important prognostic tests that determine eligibility for liver transplantation. Always discuss the situation with a liver transplant centre before administering clotting factors to a patient with acute liver injury.

> **KEY POINT**
>
> • Do not attempt to correct disorders in blood coagulation without discussing the situation with a specialist transplant unit first

Assessment of renal function

Paracetamol poisoning can cause direct renal tubular damage and this may occur early in the course of the illness. It can take several weeks to resolve and patients may require renal support even when the liver has fully recovered. Patients with most other aetiologies of acute liver failure develop renal failure only when liver failure is advanced and encephalopathy has developed. Urea synthesis is impaired in acute liver failure and it is not an accurate guide to the severity of renal dysfunction. Serum creatinine levels are therefore preferred for the monitoring of renal function.

Electrolytes

Electrolyte disturbance is common in patients with acute liver injury.

• Hyponatraemia may reflect sodium depletion from vomiting.

• Hypophosphataemia can contribute to mortality and morbidity by inducing confusion and coma and should therefore be specifically sought and corrected. The causes are multifactorial including impaired renal tubular phosphate absorption and intracellular movement caused by disturbance in acid–base homeostasis.

Blood glucose

Hypoglycaemia may follow acute hepatic necrosis and can lead to impairment of consciousness before the onset of encephalopathy. Since the classic signs and symptoms of hypoglycaemia may be masked in acute liver injury, regular blood glucose monitoring is required.

Liver function tests

Deranged liver function tests are common following paracetamol overdose but do not correlate with prognosis. Transaminases can rise into the thousands, indicating hepatic necrosis, but this gives no indication of the ability of the liver to function.

Arterial blood gas

• Metabolic acidosis is associated with acute liver failure after a paracetamol overdose and is associated with a particularly high mortality (>90% if the arterial blood pH is <7.30 more than 24 hours following the overdose).

• Hyperlactataemia is frequent following paracetamol overdose. An elevated lactate 15 hours after an overdose is an ominous sign associated with a poor prognosis. The presence of an increased lactate at this stage should prompt discussion with a liver transplant centre.

Chronic liver disease evaluation

If there is evidence of liver failure it is important to consider whether the patient might already have a coexisting chronic liver disease since this can alter their prognosis and invalidate the use of some markers for prognosis. Blood tests should be sent to look for evidence of chronic viral hepatitis, autoimmune liver disease and metabolic disorders. A liver ultrasound is required to look for features of cirrhosis such as splenomegaly, ascites or the presence of a small liver with an irregular margin. The latter finding needs to be interpreted with caution, however, since acute necrosis of hepatic parenchyma can cause the liver to appear irregular and shrunken, similar to that seen in cirrhosis.

How does paracetamol cause liver damage?

Paracetamol itself is not directly hepatotoxic. Paracetamol is converted to a toxic metabolite, N-acetyl-p-benzoquionimine (NAPQI) (Fig. 5.2). This is normally inactivated by conjugation with reduced glutathione. After a large overdose, glutathione is depleted from hepatocytes and the toxic metabolite binds covalently with sulphydryl groups on liver cell membranes leading to hepatocyte necrosis.

What are the clinical features of paracetamol overdose?

In the first 24 hours the patient may be asymptomatic or have mild symptoms such as nausea, vomiting and epigastric pain. Unless the overdose is mixed with other substances the patient is usually fully conscious in this first 24 hours. This can sometimes lead the patient to think that the overdose has not caused damage and may delay presentation to medical services. Liver failure does not usually become apparent until 72–96 hours after the overdose by which time hepatic necrosis has already occurred and the specific antidote has limited efficacy.

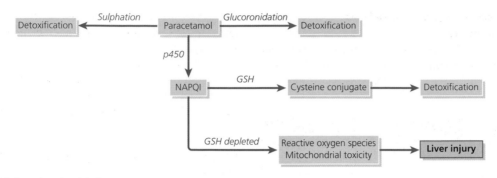

Figure 5.2 Paracetamol metabolism.

Outline the steps involved in managing a patient with suspected paracetamol overdose

The initial principles of treating a patient presenting with a paracetamol overdose are to determine the timing of the overdose if possible and to assess whether the level of paracetamol in the blood is likely to cause harm (using the normogram in Fig. 5.1). The lower line is used for high-risk patients, including those who regularly consume excess alcohol, patients taking enzyme-inducing drugs (e.g. antiepileptics) and patients who are malnourished.

If there is a risk of hepatotoxicity the specific antidote should be given (Box 5.1). The antidote of choice is *N*-acetyl cysteine, which is given by intravenous infusion. It acts to increase the availability of glutathione by producing sulphydryl groups. If treatment is started within 8 hours of suspected overdose then it is usually possible to prevent serious hepatotoxicity. Treatment started at later time points is still likely to be beneficial. *N*-acetyl cysteine treatment can occasionally cause a hypersensitivity reaction including rash, bronchospasm and hypotension. If this occurs the treatment should be stopped and the patient given treatment with intravenous hydrocortisone and chlorpheniramine. Once the reaction has subsided the infusion can be restarted at a lower rate. If this is not tolerated then oral methionine can be given as an alternative. It is effective but absorption is unreliable if the patient is vomiting.

> **Box 5.1 Management of a patient presenting with a paracetamol overdose**
>
> - Treatment depends on the interval between the overdose and the time of presentation to hospital:
>   - if the patient presents within 4 hours of ingestion and >7.5 g of paracetamol has been taken, gastric lavage should be considered or activated charcoal given to reduce absorption
>   - if 4–8 hours have elapsed since the overdose, blood should be taken and sent for paracetamol level
>   - if 8–24 hours have elapsed since the overdose, treatment should be started immediately whilst awaiting the results of blood levels. If the concentration of paracetamol is subsequently found to be below the treatment level therapy can be discontinued
> - If at 24 hours the patient is well, the INR is normal and the paracetamol level is <10 mg/L, then *N*-acetyl cysteine infusion can be discontinued. If any of these are abnormal, continue the *N*-acetyl cysteine infusion
> - *N*-acetyl cysteine should be given without the guidance of the treatment graph (Fig. 5.1) in the following situations:
>   - where the timing of the overdose is unknown
>   - where the overdose is staggered
>   - if a patient presents with evidence of severe toxicity or fulminant hepatic failure regardless of the time of the overdose

The clinical suspicion is that she has taken a significant paracetamol overdose and N-acetyl cysteine is started immediately. A few hours later she becomes increasingly restless wandering around the ward and pulling out her intravenous infusion. Further blood tests are taken and the results are as follows:

Bilirubin	*217 μmol/L*
ALT	*4316 iU/L*
ALP	*185 iU/L*
INR	*4.3*
Creatinine	*256 μmol/L*

What are the main priorities of care now?

She has liver failure as evidenced by encephalopathy and coagulopathy. She should be referred to a specialist unit with facilities for liver transplantation (Box 5.2).

Box 5.2 Criteria for transfer to a specialist liver unit

Patients with any of the features listed below should be referred immediately to a liver transplant unit:
- INR > 2.0 less than 48 hours after overdose or INR > 3.5 less than 72 hours after overdose
- Renal impairment (creatinine >200 μmol/L)
- Acidosis (pH < 7.3 or lactic acidosis unresponsive to fluid resuscitation)
- Any sign of encephalopathy
- Evidence of raised intracranial hypertension (BP > 160/90 mmHg, bradycardia, hyperreflexia, extensor spasms, poor pupil responses)

Patients with milder abnormalities should also be discussed as they may deteriorate fast and there may be only a matter of hours to obtain a donor liver for them. Furthermore, it is dangerous to transfer a patient once they have developed cardiovascular instability and cerebral oedema. If in doubt always discuss cases of severe paracetamol overdose with a specialist liver unit.

How do you manage a patient with acute liver failure?

- Patients should be managed in an intensive care unit and should be in a specialist centre that is used to looking after patients with liver failure and can consider liver transplantation if appropriate.
- Patients often have disturbed conscious levels and may require intubation and ventilation.
- Supportive care is required to maintain fluid balance, monitor and correct electrolyte disturbances, and to maintain glycaemic control.
- Renal failure is common and patients may require renal support in the form of haemofiltration.
- Cerebral oedema is the major cause of death. If signs of raised intracranial pressure develop, patients should be given mannitol intravenously as an osmotic diuretic. This treatment necessitates that the patient is passing urine; if they are not then fluid should be removed during haemofiltration.

- Infection may be a problem and patients should be given prophylactic broad spectrum antibiotic and anti-fungal agents.
- It is difficult to judge which patients will require liver transplantation and to time the procedure. National guidelines have been developed that determine which patients with acute liver failure can be offered liver transplantation.*

What other causes of acute liver failure do you know?

- *Seronegative hepatitis*: Although this is a diagnosis of exclusion it is in fact the second commonest cause of acute liver failure in the UK, with middle-aged females the most frequently affected. By definition patients have negative serology tests for viral hepatitis and autoimmune liver disease. Liver failure develops more slowly than in patients who have taken a paracetamol overdose (over 5–12 weeks) but the prospect of recovery is lower and otherwise eligible patients need to be considered for liver transplantation.
- *Acute infection with a hepatitis virus*: Acute liver failure is an uncommon outcome of viral infection of the liver, occurring in <1% of cases.
- *Autoimmune hepatitis*: This may present as acute liver failure. It is usually not amenable to treatment with immunosuppressive agents and patients should be considered for liver transplantation.
- *Drug-induced liver injury*: Many drugs other than paracetamol can cause acute liver failure (Box 5.3).
- *Pregnancy-induced liver failure*: Acute liver failure is a rare complication of pregnancy (see Case 9).
- *Wilson's disease*: This is exceptionally rare but it may present with acute liver failure, usually during the second decade of life. The prognosis is extremely poor and patients should be considered for liver transplantation.
- *Budd–Chiari syndrome*: Acute occlusion of the hepatic veins (Budd–Chiari syndrome) may present with acute liver failure. Patients usually have abdominal pain, hepatomegaly and ascites.
- *Malignant infiltration of the liver*: It is important to exclude malignant infiltration of the liver with lymphoma, or more rarely carcinoma, as these patients are not candidates for liver transplantation.
- *Others*, e.g. ischaemic hepatitis, heat stroke or sepsis.

---

*See http://www.uktransplant.org.uk/ukt/about_transplants/organ_allocation/liver/liver_organ_sharing_principles/liver_organ_sharing_principles.jsp#b4.

Box 5.3 Drugs that cause acute liver failure

- Analgesics (e.g. paracetamol, NSAIDs)
- Anaesthetic agents (e.g. halothane, isoflurane, enflurane)
- Antituberculous agents (e.g. rifampicin, isoniazid)
- Antibiotics (e.g. sulphonamides, tetracycline)
- Antiepileptics (e.g. sodium valproate, carbamazepine, phenytoin)
- Ecstasy

Miranda becomes drowsy and requires admission to the intensive care for intubation and ventilation. She is subsequently transferred to a specialist liver unit. Over the next 24 hours she becomes anuric and requires renal

support with continuous veno-venous haemodiafiltration. Over the next few days her INR begins to improve and the rest of her liver function tests slowly recover. She requires renal support for a further 10 days but her kidneys finally recover and she is medically fit to be discharged from hospital.

What must be done before she is discharged?

Once the patient has recovered from a paracetamol overdose a psychiatric assessment is mandatory to determine the level of future suicide risk and to ensure that appropriate psychiatric treatment and follow-up is arranged. A patient who develops liver failure related to a paracetamol overdose may be in hospital for a number of weeks and it is important that the reason for admission is not forgotten once the patient has finally recovered.

CASE REVIEW

This young woman was brought to hospital with abdominal pain and vomiting following a recent relationship break-up and the development of a possible depressive illness. The history strongly suggested an attempted suicide. Her liver function tests were severely deranged with grossly elevated alanine transaminase, the most likely cause of which is paracetamol hepatotoxicity. She was treated with *N*-acetyl cysteine but developed coagulopathy, encephalopathy and renal failure and required admission to the intensive care unit and transfer to a specialist liver unit. Here her liver slowly improved and she did not require liver transplantation. Her renal failure persisted for several days but eventually she made a full recovery and was referred to the local psychiatrists.

KEY POINTS

- Paracetamol overdose is the commonest cause of acute liver failure in the United Kingdom and must be considered in any patient presenting with this clinical syndrome
- Patients are often well in the first 24–36 hours and do not develop evidence of liver failure until 2–3 days after the overdose
- Paracetamol levels are unreliable if blood is taken <4 hours or >24 hours after the overdose or if the overdose has been staggered
- Early treatment with *N*-acetyl cysteine (within 8 hours) will prevent hepatotoxicity in most cases

- In patients presenting late (>24 hours after overdose) *N*-acetyl cysteine treatment may still have benefit and should be given
- The INR or prothrombin time is an important indicator of prognosis. Before giving blood products to correct coagulation discuss the case with a liver transplant centre
- Patients with acute liver failure should be discussed with a liver transplant centre if there is coagulopathy (INR >2 at 48 hours or >3.5 at 72 hours), renal failure, acidosis or encephalopathy
- All patients who survive a paracetamol overdose must be referred for a psychiatric assessment

Hepatology: Clinical Cases Uncovered, 1st edition. © Kathryn Nash and Indra Neil Guha. Published 2011 by Blackwell Publishing Ltd.

Case 6   A 4-week-old baby with jaundice and failure to thrive

Naomi Rogers is a 4-week-old female infant who is referred for investigation by her health visitor who has noticed increasing jaundice. Naomi was born at 39 weeks' gestation after a normal pregnancy with a normal birth of 3.6 kg. She was breast fed and initially gained weight but then began to lose weight despite a good appetite. Both her parents are well and there is no family history of jaundice or liver disease.

What is the differential diagnosis of jaundice in the neonatal period?

Neonatal jaundice should be classified into causes associated with unconjugated and conjugated hyperbilirubinaemia.

Unconjugated hyperbilirubinaemia

The problem is either overproduction of bilirubin or inadequate conjugation of bilirubin. There are many causes:

• *Physiological jaundice*: About 70% of breast fed infants develop jaundice in the first week of life. It is not present at birth, peaks within 2–5 days and typically lasts for less than 3 weeks. The urine and stools are normal in colour. It is more severe in premature and low birth weight babies and tends to last longer in breast fed babies. Treatment is rarely necessary. The cause is multifactorial including increased degradation of red blood cells and immaturity of the conjugating system in the neonatal period.

• *Haemolysis*: Excess destruction of red blood cells results in unconjugated hyperbilirubinaemia. The infant may be jaundiced at birth. Causes of haemolysis that are seen in the neonatal period are given in Box 6.1.

• *Perinatal haematomas*: Haemorrhage into tissues provides an increase in the bilirubin load that may exacerbate jaundice.

• *Gilbert's syndrome*: Probable autosomal recessive disorder characterised by decreased conjugation of bilirubin. It is usually asymptomatic apart from jaundice and is often detected as an incidental finding of isolated hyperbilirubinaemia.

• *Crigler–Najjar syndrome*: Very rare disorder of bilirubin conjugation associated with high levels of unconjugated bilirubin. There is a deficiency of the bilirubin-conjugating enzyme UDP–glucoronyl transferase. Two types are recognised:

  ○ *Type 1*: autosomal recessive disorder with total absence of conjugating enzyme in the liver. Patients usually die within the first year of life unless a liver transplant is performed.

  ○ *Type 2*: Probable autosomal recessive disorder characterised by reduced activity of the conjugating enzyme. Treatment for jaundice is usually required but patients can survive into adult life.

• *Hypothyroidism*: Hyperbilirubinaemia is unconjugated but the cause is unknown.

• *Sepsis*: Infection of any site in the neonatal period can lead to unconjugated hyperbilirubinaemia and jaundice.

Box 6.1 Causes of haemolysis

- Red blood cell membrane abnormalities:
  - hereditary spherocytosis
  - hereditary elliptocytosis
- Enzyme deficiencies:
  - pyruvate kinase deficiency
  - glucose-6-phosphate dehydrogenase deficiency
- Haemoglobin disorders:
  - sickle cell disease
  - thalassaemia
- Immune-mediated haemolysis:
  - ABO or Rhesus incompatibility
  - other blood type mismatches

> **Box 6.2 Infectious causes of neonatal hepatitis**
>
> | | | | |
> |---|---|---|---|
> | • Hepatitis A | May spread in nurseries for neonates | • Congenital rubella | Jaundice may be seen in the first days of life associated with hepatosplenomegaly. Hepatitis usually resolves but can occasionally fluctuate and progressive fibrosis may develop |
> | • Hepatitis B | Develops in most babies of mothers with hepatitis B infection unless prophylactic immunisation is given. Symptomatic jaundice is uncommon | | |
> | • Hepatitis C | Transmission of active hepatitis from HCV RNA positive mothers is described but is unusual and neonates are rarely jaundiced | • Congenital syphilis | Congenital syphilis is rare but may be associated with liver involvement with jaundice and progressive fibrosis |
> | • Cytomegalovirus | Common childhood infection that may be acquired transplacentally. Often asymptomatic but hepatitis with jaundice may be seen | • Toxoplasmosis | Jaundice develops within a few hours of birth with hepatomegaly |
> | • Herpes simplex | Maternal genital herpes can be transmitted to the neonate at birth and may result in hepatitis with jaundice | | |

Conjugated hyperbilirubinaemia

The problem is due to either a process affecting the liver itself or the drainage of bile from the liver.

• *Infection*: Jaundice may be caused by primary infection of the liver or as a reaction of the immature neonatal liver to infection elsewhere. Intrauterine infection with various organisms can lead to liver infection that may present with jaundice in the neonatal period (Box 6.2).

• *Metabolic*: Many metabolic conditions are associated with conjugated hyperbilirubinaemia in neonates (Box 6.3).

• *Cholestasis*: The most important infantile cholangiopathy is biliary atresia characterised by progressive destruction of the biliary system.

> **!RED FLAG**
>
> • All cases of neonatal jaundice prolonged beyond 3 weeks should be investigated since there are many serious causes that require prompt investigation and treatment to prevent problems.

What serious brain abnormality can complicate neonatal jaundice?

High levels of unconjugated hyperbilirubinaemia in the neonatal period can damage the brain, a condition known as kernicterus. Free unconjugated bilirubin is released from albumin and crosses the immature blood–brain barrier of the neonate. In the brain, bilirubin can be deposited, particularly in the basal ganglia, causing irreversible damage. The infant may become restless or lethargic and frequently develops stiffness in the limbs and neck, twitching and convulsions. Death may occur rapidly (within 24 hours); those who survive frequently have brain damage.

Kernicterus does not occur in conjugated hyperbilirubinaemia as the conjugated form of bilirubin is unable to cross the blood–brain barrier.

> **KEY POINT**
>
> • High levels of unconjugated hyperbilirubinaemia in the neonatal period require prompt treatment to prevent severe brain damage

> **Box 6.3 Metabolic causes of conjugated hyperbilirubinaemia in neonates**
>
> • Galactosaemia
> • Alpha-1 antitrypsin deficiency
> • Tyrosinosis
> • Cystic fibrosis
> • Hereditary fructose intolerance
> • Total parenteral nutrition
> • Niemann–Pick disease

How can brain damage be prevented?

• *Phototherapy*: Controlled exposure to ultraviolet light causes isomeric changes in unconjugated bilirubin, converting it to a more polarised molecule which can be excreted without complications, thus preventing brain damage.

• *Exchange transfusion*: Removes unconjugated bilirubin from the body.

What questions should you ask to further evaluate a case of prolonged neonatal jaundice?

• *When was jaundice first noticed? How has it progressed?* Jaundice present on the first day of life is always pathological. Many other causes of jaundice start on the second or third day of life. Physiological jaundice usually peaks in the first week and then improves, disappearing by 2–3 weeks. Jaundice continuing to worsen after the third week requires prompt investigation.

• *What has happened to the colour of the urine and stool?* In unconjugated hyperbilirubinaemias the urine and stool colour are normal. Darkening of the urine and pale stools are associated with hepatic or extrahepatic causes of jaundice.

• *Is there a family history of anaemia or haemolysis?*

• *Was there any history of birth trauma, excessive bruising?*

• *Did the mother have any infections or problems during pregnancy?*

• *Are there any signs of infection in the baby?*

> Naomi's mother first noticed jaundice on the second day of life. It gradually worsened over the next 3 weeks. After birth the baby passed dark meconium stools for 24 hours following which her stools became progressively paler and the colour of her urine darkened.

What investigations should be performed?

All children with prolonged neonatal jaundice need thorough investigation (Fig. 6.1).

• *Bilirubin*: Serum bilirubin levels are a guide to the severity of the jaundice and the risk of complications. Fractionation of the bilirubin into unconjugated and conjugated forms is very important in neonates as it narrows down the differential diagnosis and allows further investigations to be targeted accordingly.

• *Liver enzymes*: Elevation in liver enzymes (ALT or alkaline phosphatase) may suggest a hepatic or extrahepatic cause for jaundice. It is important to note that alka-

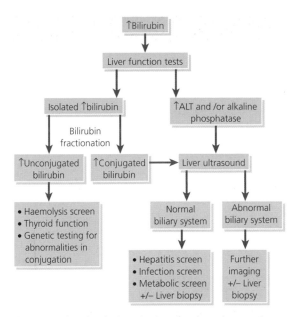

Figure 6.1 Algorithm for investigation of prolonged neonatal jaundice.

line phosphatase levels are typically elevated in the neonatal period due to bone metabolism.

• *Full blood count, blood film and haemolysis screen.*

• *Thyroid function test*: Most infants are screened for hypothyroidism in the early neonatal period but it is essential to check that this has been performed.

• *Infection screen*: Blood should be checked for IgM antibodies to toxoplasmosis, rubella, CMV and herpes simplex as well as syphilis and viral hepatitis serology. A search for systemic sources of infection should be made including blood, urine and stool culture, chest X-ray and careful examination of the umbilical stump.

• *Metabolic screen*: Blood should be sent for α_1-antitrypsin level and phenotype and a sweat test should be performed to look for cystic fibrosis. Screening for rare inborn errors of metabolism should be performed in consultation with specialists in this area.

• *Urinalysis*: High levels of urobilinogen are consistent with unconjugated hyperbilirubinaemia. High levels of bilirubin in the urine suggest a hepatic or extrahepatic cause for jaundice.

• *Liver ultrasound*: Ultrasound is necessary to define whether an extrahepatic biliary system is present and whether it has a normal appearance.

• *Biliary excretion*: Radioisotope imaging may be performed to demonstrate whether bile can be excreted from the liver into the gut.

• *Liver biopsy*: If the hyperbilirubinaemia is conjugated and neonatal infection and metabolic disorders have been excluded it may be necessary to perform a liver biopsy.

> *Investigations reveal the presence of conjugated hyperbilirubinaemia with a significantly raised alkaline phosphatase. Infection and metabolic screens are negative. Naomi has an abdominal ultrasound after a 4-hour fast which fails to demonstrate a gallbladder. A liver biopsy is performed that demonstrates expanded portal tracts with proliferation of the bile ducts and portal fibrosis.*

What is the likely diagnosis?
Extrahepatic biliary atresia.

What are the characteristics of this disorder?
Biliary atresia affects about 1 in 10 000 live births with a slight female predominance. The aetiology is unknown. It is characterised by gradual fibrosis and obliteration of the extrahepatic and intrahepatic biliary ducts. Infants are usually born at term with a normal birth weight. Jaundice begins to develop on the second day and gradually progresses, becoming associated with pale stools and dark urine. There is increasing hepatomegaly and the infant fails to gain weight despite feeding well. There may be abnormalities in other organs, e.g. congenital cardiac disorders or polysplenia.

The following abnormalities are found:
• Conjugated hyperbilirubinaemia.
• Raised alkaline phosphatase (commonly 5–10 times the upper limit of normal).
• Elevation of transaminases (2–5 times the upper limit of normal).
• An absent or small contracted gallbladder on ultrasound performed after a period of fasting.
• Absent biliary excretion from the liver on radioisotope scanning.
• Liver histology revealing expanded portal tracts, portal fibrosis and portal oedema.

What is the management?
The majority of cases are managed by a surgical procedure called a Kasai portoenterostomy (Fig. 6.2). The obliterated biliary tree is resected and a loop of small intestine is anastomosed to the proximal common hepatic duct. This can achieve biliary drainage in up to 85% of cases. The operation should be performed before

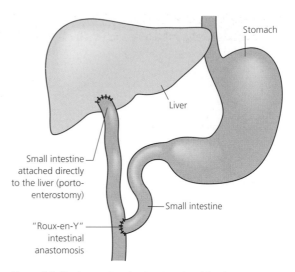

Figure 6.2 Kasai procedure (portoenterostomy) for the treatment of biliary atresia.

the infant is 2 months old; if surgery is delayed beyond this it is unlikely to be successful as the small hilar bile ducts will have disappeared. If the Kasai procedure does not result in adequate biliary drainage or there is advanced hepatic fibrosis with portal hypertension at presentation, patients should be considered for liver transplantation. Even with a successful Kasai procedure, up to 80% will require liver transplantation, but many of these can be deferred until adult life.

KEY POINT

• Surgery for biliary atresia must be performed promptly (before the infant is 2 months old) to have the best chance of achieving biliary drainage

---

> *Naomi is taken to theatre at the age of 7 weeks. An operative cholangiogram is performed which demonstrates the absence of extrahepatic biliary flow, confirming the diagnosis of biliary atresia. The surgeon performs a Kasai portoenterostomy. She initially makes good postoperative progress and her jaundice improves; 10 days following the operation her jaundice worsens again associated with fever. A diagnosis of cholangitis is suspected and she is treated with intravenous antibiotics. Her fever improves but her jaundice continues to worsen and she develops splenomegaly and ascites. She is listed for liver transplantation but unfortunately dies before a suitable donor can be found.*

CASE REVIEW

This baby was born at term with a normal birth weight. Jaundice developed on the second day of life and progressively worsened, associated with dark urine and pale stools. Investigation revealed a conjugated hyperbilirubinaemia without evidence of neonatal infection or a metabolic cause for jaundice. Ultrasound imaging failed to demonstrate an extrahepatic biliary tree suggesting a diagnosis of biliary atresia. A Kasai portoenterostomy was performed within 2 months but was complicated by cholangitis. She developed progressive liver failure and portal hypertension and died before liver transplantation could be performed.

KEY POINTS

- Most babies develop transient jaundice in the neonatal period (physiological jaundice)
- Jaundice present on the first day of life is pathological and requires investigation
- Neonatal jaundice persisting beyond 3 weeks requires investigation
- Differentiation of hyperbilirubinaemia into unconjugated and conjugated forms is essential to aid diagnosis and guide further investigation and management
- Untreated unconjugated hyperbilirubinaemia can lead to serious brain damage (kernicterus) and potential death

- Conjugated hyperbilirubinaemia should be investigated by looking for congenital infections, neonatal sepsis, metabolic causes and biliary atresia
- If surgery is performed for extrahepatic biliary atresia it must be performed before the infant is 2 months old to be successful
- Patients with failed Kasai portoenterostomy or those presenting with liver failure, portal hypertension or cirrhosis on liver biopsy should be referred to a specialised centre to be considered for liver transplantation

Case 7   A 24-year-old woman with HIV and tuberculosis develops jaundice

Janet Okecha, a 24-year-old HIV-positive Zimbabwean woman, presents to her GP with jaundice. Two months previously she was diagnosed with pulmonary tuberculosis. She had been treated in hospital for 4 weeks and established on therapy for her tuberculosis with isoniazid, rifampicin, pyrazinamide and ethambutol. Her liver function tests were normal when she was discharged from hospital. She has been taking highly active antiretroviral therapy (HAART) for HIV infection for 18 months.

Her liver function tests are as follows:

Bilirubin	165 µmol/L
ALT	325 iU/L
ALP	163 iU/L
INR	1.1

What is the most likely cause of her deranged liver function tests?

A reaction to one of the drugs used to treat tuberculosis.

What other causes should be considered?

All causes of jaundice should be considered, for example:
- Prehepatic (haemolysis, bilirubin conjugation abnormality).
- Hepatic (parenchymal liver disease).
- Posthepatic (biliary obstruction).

In a woman presenting with this set of problems there are a number of special considerations:
- *Viral hepatitis*: She comes from a part of the world where hepatitis virus infection is common, particularly hepatitis B. Furthermore, HIV shares common modes of transmission with hepatitis B and C and co-infection is frequent. Patients with viral hepatitis (both hepatitis B

and C) who are co-infected with HIV have more severe liver disease than patients without HIV infection.
- *HIV*: HIV itself can infect hepatocytes although it is unclear whether it causes direct damage to the liver. The liver is frequently involved in HIV infection, however (Box 7.1).
- *Tuberculosis*: TB itself frequently infects the liver although in most cases it is asymptomatic and jaundice is uncommon. Enlargement of liver hilar lymph nodes as a result of hepatic TB may result in jaundice by causing obstruction to bile flow.
- *Drug-related liver damage*: The drugs used to treat TB and HIV are frequently associated with abnormal liver function tests. As several drugs are used in combination it can be difficult to know which is the agent responsible. Mechanisms of HAART-related toxicity are given in Box 7.2.

What would you do?

After taking a full history and examining the patient, investigations should be undertaken to try to identify the cause of the jaundice. Even if the diagnosis appears obvious from the history it is crucial to consider all possibilities as multiple pathologies are frequent and missing a treatable co-factor such as viral hepatitis can have serious consequences. The following investigations should be performed:
- Viral hepatitis serology.
- Immunoglobulins and liver autoantibody screen.
- Metabolic screen (ferritin, caeruloplasmin, α_1-antitrypsin level).
- Evaluation of conjugated and unconjugated bilirubin to assess whether there is a prehepatic component to the jaundice.
- Liver ultrasound.

Further investigation will be dictated by the results of the above investigations. Figure 7.1 illustrates an algorithm for the investigation of abnormal liver function tests in HIV infection.

Hepatology: Clinical Cases Uncovered, 1st edition. © Kathryn Nash and Indra Neil Guha. Published 2011 by Blackwell Publishing Ltd.

ally lead to liver failure. The latter case is rare but associated with a high mortality and the drug must be stopped.
- *Rifampicin*: Liver injury occurs in less than 5% of people taking rifampicin. Hepatotoxicity is more common when rifampicin is given in combination with isoniazid due to its ability to induce drug-metabolising systems within the hepatocytes.
- *Pyrazinamide*: Hepatotoxicity is occasionally seen.

What changes to her medication would you make?

The first step is to stop all antituberculous drugs. The most likely cause of hepatotoxicity is isoniazid followed by rifampicin and finally pyrazinamide. It is not possible to tell which of these agents is injurious, however, so it is essential that all are stopped. Ethambutol is regarded as a non-hepatotoxic agent; however it should never be given as monotherapy due to the risks of developing TB resistance.

She has had inadequate treatment for her TB infection and is going to need further treatment. TB can rapidly become resistant if treated with single agents, therefore there is no place for starting one drug at a time to see if it is tolerated. Alternative non-hepatotoxic regimens can be given (e.g. ethambutol, streptomycin and a quinolone antibiotic such as moxifloxacin).

Once liver function tests have returned to normal, the original drugs can be reintroduced sequentially, initially at low dose and increasing as tolerated to the normal treatment dose. If there is no further reaction standard drugs can be continued and the alternative drugs that were introduced temporarily can be withdrawn. If there is a further reaction the offending drug can be withdrawn and an alternative substituted.

Managing drug-induced liver disease in TB infection is very difficult and requires a multidisciplinary approach involving a hepatologist and TB physician.

Isoniazid, rifampicin and pyrazinamide treatment are discontinued. She continues on ethambutol and additional therapy with streptomycin and moxifloxacin is added. Over the next 2 weeks her liver function tests settle back to normal. Isoniazid is restarted at a low dose but the ALT rises again 2 days later and the isoniazid is discontinued. Rifampicin and pyrazinamide are gradually reintroduced without any change in the liver function tests. This allows the streptomycin to be discontinued and she is discharged home on quadruple therapy with ethambutol, rifampicin, moxifloxacin and pyrazinamide.

Box 7.1 Hepatobiliary involvement with HIV infection

Non-specific effects of HIV infection
- Hepatomegaly
- Abnormal liver biochemistry
- Histological changes, e.g. steatosis, portal inflammation

Opportunistic infections
- Mycobacteria (e.g. *Mycobacterium tuberculosis*, *M. avium-intracellulare*, *M. kansaii*)
- Viruses (e.g. cytomegalovirus, herpes simplex virus, Epstein–Barr virus)
- Fungal infection (e.g. *Cryptococcus neoformans*, hepatic candidiasis, histoplasmosis)
- Protozoal infection (e.g. toxoplasmosis, cryptosporidium, *Pneumocystis jirovecii* (previously known as *P. carinii*))

Neoplasms
- Lymphoma (Hodgkin's or non-Hodgkin's)
- Kaposi's sarcoma (rare)

Box 7.2 Mechanisms of HAART-related changes in liver blood tests

- Isolated hyperbilirubinaemia due to interference with bilirubin conjugation (e.g. indinavir)
- Hepatocyte toxicity (e.g. ritonavir)
- Cholestatic reaction (e.g. nevaripine)
- Mitochondrial toxicity producing steatosis (e.g. didanosine, stavudine)
- Hypersensitivity reactions (e.g. abacavir)

The blood results exclude viral hepatitis and other causes of acute and chronic hepatitis. The liver ultrasound is normal. Her medication is reviewed, the HIV medication, although associated with hepatotoxicity, has not been changed for 18 months and she had normal liver function tests throughout this time. It is therefore considered most likely that it is the new medication for TB which has caused the problem.

Which drugs used to treat TB are associated with hepatotoxicity?

Most of the antituberculous drugs can cause hepatotoxicity in susceptible individuals. Drugs that are commonly associated with liver pathology are:
- *Isoniazid*: This is a common cause of hepatotoxicity. Liver damage ranges from a mild hepatitis, which occurs in up to 20% of users and resolves despite continuation of the drug, to hepatocyte necrosis, which can occasion-

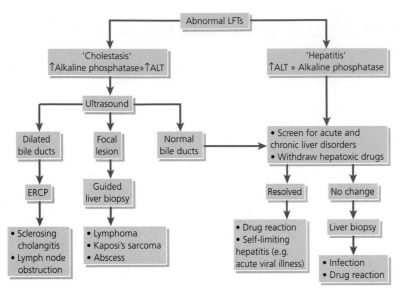

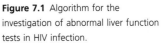

Figure 7.1 Algorithm for the investigation of abnormal liver function tests in HIV infection.

CASE REVIEW

This young woman has HIV infection which is stable on HAART. She developed abnormal liver function tests and jaundice shortly after starting treatment for TB. She underwent investigation which excluded prehepatic and posthepatic pathology. Her liver disease screen was normal making drug toxicity the most likely cause. All the hepa-totoxic antituberculous agents were stopped and she was established on alternative agents. Once her liver function tests had normalised the original drugs were reintroduced although isoniazid was not tolerated and it was likely that it was a reaction to this agent that caused her liver disease.

KEY POINTS

- Patients may have multiple reasons for developing abnormal liver biochemistry; all possible causes should be considered even if the history is suggestive of one particular cause
- HIV infection can result in many different effects on the liver, particularly opportunistic infections, tumours and toxicity related to HIV therapy
- Antituberculous therapy is frequently associated with derangement in liver function tests

- In drug-induced liver injury it is vital to take a careful history eliciting all recent and past drug exposure (including non-prescribed agents)
- It is important to stop all potentially hepatotoxic agents
- Patients with TB should not be treated with single agent therapy due to the risk of developing drug resistance

Case 8 Abnormal liver function tests in a collapsed patient

You are on call during an evening shift and asked to review a patient on the care of the elderly ward. The staff nurses have been phoned by the biochemistry department with some very abnormal blood results and they are extremely concerned. The blood tests are as follows:

Bilirubin	*120 μmol/L*
ALT	*986 iU/L*
ALP	*108 iU/L*
AST	*689 iU/L*
INR	*1.6*
Renal function	*Normal*
Full blood count	*Normal*

On reading though the medical notes and speaking to the patient you gather the following history: Mr Darren Williams is an 82-year-old man who was admitted with a collapse the day before. He has little recollection of the collapse and this has never occurred previously. He has little medical history of note and is usually independent and self-caring. There is no history of liver disease and he is teetotal. On examination he looks well with a blood pressure of 120/90 mmHg and pulse of 80 beats per minute. He is jaundiced but there are no signs of chronic liver disease. The medical team managing his care have performed a number of tests for his collapse, including:
ECG: atrial fibrillation but no acute ischaemic changes
Troponin at 12 hours was normal
CK >1000 iU/L
CT head: no evidence of an acute ischaemic event or intracerebral bleed

What are the main differential diagnoses that you should consider?
• Ischaemic hepatitis (Box 8.1).
• Sepsis (Box 8.2).

Hepatology: Clinical Cases Uncovered, 1st edition. © Kathryn Nash and Indra Neil Guha. Published 2011 by Blackwell Publishing Ltd.

• Paracetamol overdose. An unexplained transaminitis should always trigger the possibility of a paracetamol overdose. Measuring paracetamol levels at this stage of the admission are not helpful but measuring levels in the serum at initial presentation is useful.
• Acute viral hepatitis. There are no major risk factors in the history but this a diagnosis that needs to be excluded.

On review of the observation charts from the emergency department there is documented hypotension when he arrived the previous day. Collateral history from a neighbour confirms that he had collapsed for an extended period of time. Over the next 72 hours he remains stable. His liver function tests improve to normal by day 5 of his admission (Fig. 8.1).

His viral serological tests are normal and paracetamol levels are undetectable on initial serum taken in the emergency department. He is awaiting a liver ultrasound. The medical team are planning to commence him on anticoagulation and discharge him when he suddenly develops central chest pain. An ECG shows new ST elevation in the inferior leads. He is transferred to the acute coronary care unit and given intravenous thrombolysis. A troponin level confirms an ST elevation myocardial infarction (STEMI) and Mr Williams is managed as an acute coronary syndrome using the standard protocol. A day after his myocardial infarction he is noted to be jaundiced. On examination he has an elevated jugular venous pressure and a tender liver edge. His liver function tests which had become normal are now markedly elevated.

What is the diagnosis?
The likely diagnosis is right-sided heart failure; it is probable that he has right ventricular dysfunction (an inferior myocardial infarction) which has caused acute congestive liver failure. The liver failure is caused by a combination of 'backward' failure due to high venous pressure but also 'forward' failure because the right side of heart is unable

Box 8.1 Hepatic ischaemia

- The liver is relatively protected from ischaemia due to its receiving blood from both the portal vein and hepatic artery
- During prolonged hypotension the liver is at risk of ischaemia particularly if this occurs in the presence of hypoxia and/or 'backward failure' from congestive heart failure
- The clinical presentation is often silent and considered only when there are highly deranged liver function tests in the presence of an acute cardiac event or circulatory collapse
- The patency of the hepatic artery and portal vein should be considered in cases of hepatic ischaemia
- Depending on the aetiology, ischemic hepatitis is usually self-limiting. The liver function tests may worsen in the following days after the insult before improving to normal with conservative management
- The diagnosis is a clinical one based on the findings above and exclusion of other causes of acute hepatitis. If a liver biopsy is performed, in cases where there is diagnostic doubt, it will reveal centrilobular necrosis
- Careful observation is required for the complications of acute liver failure that may accompany ischaemia

Box 8.2 Relationship between sepsis and the liver

- Sepsis can cause a non-specific derangement in liver function tests. This may be related to sepsis within the liver (e.g. hepatic abscesses), the biliary system (e.g. cholangitis) or a generalised septicaemia
- In severe sepsis the associated circulatory collapse may precipitate an ischaemic hepatitis, especially in the presence of underlying cardiac dysfunction
- Features of sepsis including a tachycardia, fever, raised white cell count and elevated CRP will often initiate the search for a source, but in the elderly they may not be pronounced

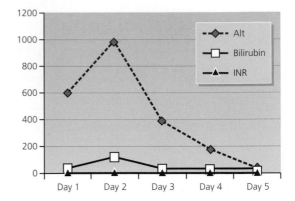

Figure 8.1 Liver function tests following an episode of ischaemic hepatitis in this patient.

Box 8.3 Associations of the heart and liver

Examples of aetiological agents causing direct damage to the heart and liver
- Alcohol
- Iron
- Amyloid

Examples of cardiac disease causing liver dysfunction
- Acute cardiac failure
- Chronic cardiac failure
- Tricuspid regurgitation
- Constrictive pericarditis

Examples of drugs for cardiac disease causing liver dysfunction
- Enalapril and methyldopa (acute hepatitis)
- Atenolol and hydralzine (cholestasis)
- Diltiazem and quinidine (granulomatous hepatitis)
- Amiodarone (non-alcoholic steatohepatitis)

to deliver a sufficient volume of blood to the systemic circulation. Treatment of the underling cardiac dysfunction will improve the liver dysfunction. The heart and liver are linked by a number of conditions shown in Box 8.3.

What pathological changes are seen in the liver in right heart failure?

Congestion of the liver results in dilated hepatic venules which appear as dark spots surrounded by paler unaffected liver. The pathological appearance is likened to a nutmeg kernel (Fig. 8.2). If congestion is severe and long-standing it can lead to fibrosis when it is referred to as cardiac cirrhosis.

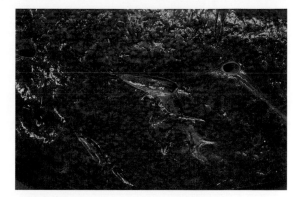

Figure 8.2 Macroscopic photograph of a liver showing marked venous congestion.

CASE REVIEW

An 82-year-old man is admitted with a collapse of unknown cause. He has asymptomatic hepatitis. On review of his previous observations there is documented hypotension. The working diagnosis is ischaemic hepatitis and his liver function tests improve with conservative manage-ment. During his admission he has an acute coronary event and develops right-sided heart failure. This is associated with liver congestion and a further episode of liver dysfunction.

KEY POINTS

- The dual blood supply of the liver offers greater protection form ischaemic events. However, prolonged hypotension in the presence of cardiac dysfunction and/or hypoxia can lead to ischaemia
- Sepsis and other causes of acute liver failure need to be considered as important differentials for ischaemic hepatitis
- Ischaemic hepatitis is usually a self-limiting condition depending on correction of the precipitating aetiology
- There are a number of associations between the liver and heart

Case 9 Abnormal liver function tests in a pregnant woman

Mrs Jane Okegwu is a 34-year-old Nigerian history teacher. She presents to her midwife with symptoms of nausea and right upper quadrant discomfort. She is 36 weeks' pregnant and this is her first pregnancy. There is no past medical history of note. She is currently teetotal and was drinking less than 10 units of alcohol before becoming pregnant. The midwife documents her blood pressure to be 110/60mmHg and pulse 80 beats per minute. She checks some blood tests and calls you for advice:

Bilirubin	*50 µmol/L*
ALT	*198 iU/L*
ALP	*398 iU/L*
Albumin	*28 g/L*
Urea	*1.2 mmol/L*
Creatinine	*76 µmol/L*
Hb	*10.3 g/dL*
WBC	*6.8 × 10⁹/L*
Plt	*110 × 10⁹/L*
PT	*12 seconds*
AFP	*30 iU/mL*

Which of these values should concern you?

The normal physiological changes of pregnancy result in an increased cardiac output in the third trimester. Due to the vasodilatation, the blood pressure will actually fall in the second trimester before returning to normal at term. There is a fall in serum albumin, urea, total protein and the haematocrit. ALP and AFP increase in normal pregnancy (produced by the placenta). Therefore the blood tests above that cannot be explained by a normal pregnancy are the low platelet count and elevated bilirubin and ALT.

What specific aspects of the history and examination are pertinent in this case?

Liver disease in the context of pregnancy can be divided into:

1 Diseases caused by the pregnancy (Table 9.1).
2 Diseases unrelated to pregnancy but occurring during pregnancy.
3 Patients with established liver disease who become pregnant.

The purpose of the history, examination and investigations are to try and disentangle these possibilities. The broad principles of investigating abnormal liver tests should be employed with specific attention to the following areas.

History

• *Previous liver disease*: Check if there is a history of previous liver disease.
• *Hepatitis B status*: This is routinely ascertained in the antenatal period during the first trimester and should be looked for in the obstetric notes. If she is known to have chronic hepatitis B this will have been flagged (the newborn will need treatment with immunoglobulin and subsequent vaccination to reduce vertical transmission) and the possibility of reactivation will need to be excluded.
• *Drug history*: Pay specific attention to herbal remedies and antibiotics (tetracycline can induce fatty liver of pregnancy).
• *Foreign travel*: Hepatitis A and E are responsible for a significant numbers of maternal deaths from fulminant liver failure in developing countries. Travel to endemic regions should be asked about.
• *History of pruritus and family history*: She is not complaining of pruritus but this should be specifically enquired about as it may indicate intrahepatic cholestasis of pregnancy (ICP). ICP is associated with genetic mutations, so a family history of pruritus of pregnancy is

Hepatology: Clinical Cases Uncovered, 1st edition. © Kathryn Nash and Indra Neil Guha. Published 2011 by Blackwell Publishing Ltd.

Table 9.1 Liver diseases specific to pregnancy.

Condition	Timing	Symptoms	Blood tests	Notes
Acute fatty liver of pregnancy	Third trimester	Right upper quadrant pain, nausea and vomiting	Raised AST/ALT Raised bilirubin Heamolysis screen can be positive	Risk of liver failure Management by urgent delivery of the baby
Pre-eclampsia	Second/third trimester	Right upper quadrant pain, nausea, vomiting, headaches and oedema	Raised AST/ALT Bilirubin normal Uric acid raised DIC in severe cases	Increased maternal mortality Management by urgent delivery of the baby
HELLP (haemolysis, elevated liver enzymes, low platelet count)	Second/third trimester	Right upper quadrant pain, nausea and vomiting	Raised AST/ALT Raised bilirubin Low platelets Haemolysis screen positive	Increased maternal and fetal mortality
Intrahepatic cholestasis	Second/third trimester	Itching Risk of stillbirth therefore fetus may be delivered at 37 weeks	Raised AST/ALT Raised ALP Raised bilirubin Raised bile acids	Increased risk of stillbirth Management by improving bile flow with ursodeoxycholic acid and delivery as soon as the fetus is mature (around 37 weeks' gestation)
Hyperemesis gravidarum	First trimester	Vomiting	Raised AST/ALT Raised bilirubin	Associated with low birth weight

ALP, alkaline phosphatase; ALT, alanine aminotransferase; AST, aspartate aminotransferase; DIC, disseminated intravascular coagulopathy.

relevant. Furthermore, episodes of pruritus during menstruation or use of the oral contraceptive pill may suggest ICP or signify benign recurrent intrahepatic cholestasis (BRIC) which is associated with ICP.

Investigations
• Chronic liver disease screen (viral serology, autoantibodies, metabolic screen).
• Acute viral infections including hepatitis A, E and B, HSV, EBV and CMV.
• If there has been foreign travel further viral serology will be needed depending on the area of travel.
• Pregnancy-related liver disease:
  ○ Check urine for proteinuria
  ○ Haemolysis screen and blood film
  ○ Uric acid
  ○ Bile acids.
• *Imaging*: Ultrasound has no implications for the foetus. With modern CT scans the radiation exposure is reduced due to rapid acquisition times. As this is the

third trimester, the diagnostic benefit will often outweigh the risks.
• *Liver biopsy*: The risk of liver biopsy is not increased in pregnancy but it is reserved for cases of diagnostic uncertainty and when it will change imminent management.

Mrs Okegwu has no history of liver disease. She is hepatitis B surface antigen negative. There is no history of foreign travel, recent antibiotics or family history. A liver screen (including viral serology) is sent for. There is very mild proteinuria, the haemolysis screen is negative and the blood film shows a neutophilia with giant platelets. An urgent abdominal ultrasound reveals steatosis and patency of the normal hepatic vasculature. Following discussion between the consultant obstetrician and consultant hepatologist, an urgent CT scan of the abdomen is arranged. This reveals marked steatosis and a small subcapsular haemorrhage but no rupture of the liver.

What is the likely diagnosis and what should the management plan be:

This woman has presented in the third trimester with symptoms and radiological features of an acute fatty liver of pregnancy (Box 9.1). The other major differentials include pre-eclampsia and the HELLP syndrome (a condition characterised by *h*eamolysis, *e*levated *l*iver enzymes and *l*ow *p*latelets). The management of all of these conditions involves delivery of the baby.

Mrs Okegwu has an emergency caesarean section. The baby requires one night on the special care baby unit and then makes an excellent recovery. Following delivery, Mrs Okegwu's liver returns to normal and follow-up imaging shows resolution of the steatosis and haemorrhage.

Box 9.1 Acute fatty liver of pregnancy (AFLP)

- Usually occurs in the third trimester of pregnancy
- Pathology lies in an enzyme defect in the foetus (long chain hydroxyacyl coenzyme A, which metabolises fatty acids). If the mother is also heterozygote, she is unable to metabolise the excess free fatty acids and these are subsequently deposited in the liver
- Symptoms include nausea, vomiting and right upper quadrant pain
- CT imaging is often required because of the associated risk of liver haematomas, haemorrhage and rupture
- Liver biopsy, if performed, will show microvesicular steatosis and there is often little inflammation or necrosis

- There is a risk of fulminant liver failure, renal failure, disseminated intravascular coagulation, pancreatitis and fetal mortality
- Will only resolve by delivery of the fetus
- If liver haemorrhage occurs, this is ideally managed conservatively but needs very careful observation because of the risk of liver rupture. If this occurs, hepatic surgery is required and in a minority of cases a liver transplant is needed as well
- There is a close association between AFLP and other pregnancy-induced liver disease, in particular HELLP syndrome and pre-eclampsia. In clinical practice they can be difficult to distinguish and it may be that they are best thought of as a spectrum of disease

---

CASE REVIEW

A 34-year-old teacher presents to her midwife, with nausea and right upper quadrant discomfort, in the third trimester of pregnancy. Blood tests show a low platelet count and elevated bilirubin and ALT. The liver screen, including hepatitis B, is negative. Imaging, including ultrasound and CT, show marked steatosis in the liver and a subcapsular haemorrhage. A diagnosis of acute fatty liver of pregnancy is made and the baby is delivered by emergency caesarean section. Resolution of the mother's clinical symptoms and biochemistry occurs after delivery.

KEY POINTS

- Liver dysfunction in pregnancy can be classified into three broad areas: (i) diseases caused by the pregnancy; (ii) diseases unrelated to pregnancy but occurring during pregnancy; and (iii) patients with established liver disease who become pregnant.
- Normal physiological changes in pregnancy cause alterations in baseline blood tests including: albumin, urea, heamatocrit, AFP and ALP
- The timing of the pregnancy can give clues to the aetiology of disease

- Investigations such as a haemolysis screen, bile acids and proteinuria are important tests in pregnancy-related dysfunction
- Imaging can be helpful in aiding diagnosis and excluding complications such as rupture of the liver, particularly in the third trimester
- Liver diseases specific to pregnancy can have similar features and may be difficult to separate clinically
- Delivery of the baby will improve maternal and fetal wellbeing in acute fatty liver of pregnancy, HELLP and pre-eclampsia

Case 10   A 27-year-old woman with abdominal pain and distension

Zöe Clements is a 27-year-old secretary who is normally fit and well. She presents to hospital with a 3-week history of nausea, vomiting and increasing abdominal distension associated with pain in the upper abdomen. She reports no past medical history and her only medication is the oral contraceptive pill. Her mother had a history of deep venous thromboses and a pulmonary embolus and was maintained on long-term anticoagulation. Zöe smokes 10 cigarettes a day and drinks 30 units of alcohol a week.

On examination she is uncomfortable and clearly in pain. There are no signs of chronic liver disease and no evidence of encephalopathy. Cardiovascular and respiratory examinations are normal. Her liver is palpable and very tender and there is marked abdominal distension with shifting dullness consistent with ascites. Blood tests are as follows:

Bilirubin	*30 μmol/L*
ALT	*97 iU/L*
ALP	*48 iU/L*
Albumin	*36 g/L*
INR	*1.5*
Full blood count	*Normal*
Urea and creatinine	*Normal*

Give a differential diagnosis for her presentation

She was previously well but has rapidly developed ascites with deranged liver function tests. This is most likely caused by an acute event, for example:

• *Acute liver injury*: Acute damage to the liver (e.g. by viruses or drugs) could account for her becoming rapidly unwell with deranged liver function tests. Mild abdominal pain is sometimes a feature of acute liver injury. Whilst some ascites may form, the rapid development of large volume ascites would be uncommon in an acute liver parenchymal injury.

• *Vascular event*: Thrombosis of the hepatic venous system obstructs blood flow out of the liver, leading to painful hepatic congestion and ascites. Portal vein thrombosis produces abdominal pain which may be associated with gastrointestinal symptoms such as diarrhoea. In patients with underlying cirrhosis or intra-abdominal malignancy, the development of portal vein thrombosis may cause ascites production.

• *Pancreatitis*: Acute pancreatitis is a cause of abdominal pain with ascites production.

• *Inferior vena cava obstruction*: Obstruction of the inferior vena cava (e.g. by thrombosis or intra-abdominal malignancy) may cause rapid development of ascites. Oedema of the lower limbs is often a prominent feature.

• *Cardiac disorders*: Right-sided heart failure or pericardial constriction may cause prominent ascites and hepatic congestion.

What would you do?

This patient is unwell and requires urgent investigation:

• *Serum amylase*: Pancreatitis should be considered in anyone presenting with an acute abdomen.

• *Arterial blood gases*: Metabolic derangement should be sought for by performing arterial blood gases looking specifically for an acidosis or elevation in lactate levels.

• *Abdominal ultrasound with Doppler investigation*: She should have radiological imaging to assess liver size and echotexture, to look for signs of underlying cirrhosis (nodular liver with irregular margin, splenomegaly) and to assess the intra-abdominal vasculature. Views of the pancreas may be obtained but often this organ is obscured by gas in the overlying bowel.

• *Ascitic fluid analysis*: A sample of ascitic fluid should be sent for biochemistry (protein, LDH, amylase), microscopy and culture and for cytological examination.

Hepatology: Clinical Cases Uncovered, 1st edition. © Kathryn Nash and Indra Neil Guha. Published 2011 by Blackwell Publishing Ltd.

• *Echocardiogram*: An echocardiogram should be considered to assess cardiac function and to look for pericardial disease.

> Her serum amylase was normal. Ultrasound examination confirmed large volume ascites. The spleen size was normal. The liver was enlarged but of normal echotexture with a smooth margin. The portal vein was patent with normal flow but there was no flow in the hepatic veins, which appeared distended.

What is the diagnosis?

Hepatic venous outlet obstruction (Box 10.1). Obstruction can arise at any site between the parenchymal central veins and the inferior vena cava (IVC). Obstruction of the hepatic venules may be called venoocclusive disease and obstruction of the main hepatic veins may be called the Budd–Chiari syndrome. In the majority of cases obstruction is caused by thrombosis but other causes such as tumour invasion or fibrotic webs may occur.

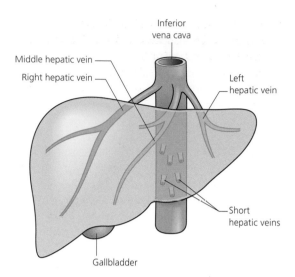

Figure 10.1 Venous drainage of the liver.

Box 10.1 Causes of hepatic venous outlet obstruction

- Myeloproliferative disorder (associated in up to 60% of cases)
- Coagulopathy (e.g. factor V Leiden mutation, deficiency of protein C, protein S or antithrombin III, anticardiolipin antibody, etc.)
- Drugs (e.g. oral contraceptive pill)
- Pregnancy
- Malignancy (e.g. hepatocellular carcinoma, renal cell carcinoma, adrenal carcinoma)
- Inferior vena cava web
- Infection (e.g. schistosomiasis, amoebic liver abscess)
- Abdominal trauma
- Abdominal radiotherapy
- Idiopathic causes

Describe the venous drainage of the liver

The liver is drained by three main veins, the right, middle and left hepatic veins. These veins drain into the IVC just below the diaphragm (Fig. 10.1). Short hepatic veins drain the posterior surface of the liver (caudate lobe) directly into the IVC and are usually spared in hepatic venous outflow obstruction, allowing the caudate lobe to become hypertrophic.

How do patients with hepatic venous outflow obstruction present?

The classic clinical presentation is with the triad of abdominal pain, hepatomegaly and ascites. The time course of the presentation may vary:
• Fulminant hepatic failure develops over a few days. This is a rare presentation; patients develop jaundice and rapidly progress to coma and death.
• The acute form develops over a few weeks. Patients are unwell with abdominal pain, nausea, vomiting, tender hepatomegaly and rapid development of ascites.
• The chronic form develops over many months. Ascites is the classic feature; this may be resistant to medical management and may be associated with renal impairment. Hepatomegaly may be present with the caudate lobe in particular being enlarged. The caudate lobe drains venous blood independently into the IVC so it may not be involved in the venous obstruction and can develop compensatory hypertrophy. Patients with chronic venous outflow obstruction may develop gastrointestinal haemorrhage and splenomegaly.

KEY POINT

- Always consider the possibility of acute hepatic venous outflow obstruction in a patient presenting with painful hepatomegaly and ascites

What investigations should be performed in suspected hepatic venous outflow obstruction?

Investigations need to consider both diagnosing hepatic venous outflow obstruction and, in addition, investigating the possible cause.

Diagnosis

• Ultrasound can diagnose hepatic venous outflow obstruction in up to 75% of cases. Echogenic material may be seen in the hepatic veins or there may be a visible stenosis of the veins with proximal dilatation.

• CT and MRI may be useful if the ultrasound is not diagnostic. They may provide additional information, e.g. demonstrating caudate lobe hypertrophy.

• Hepatic venography may be performed by retrograde cannulation of the hepatic veins from the IVC. It is of value in diagnosis and may be important in aiding treatment decision making.

• Liver biopsy is not necessary in many cases as the diagnosis may be obvious from the radiological imaging. If undertaken, the classic feature is centrilobular congestion. Patients with the chronic form may no longer show congestion if they have progressed to cirrhosis.

Aetiology

• The most common causes of hepatic vein occlusion are myeloproliferative disorders and hypercoagulable states, therefore patients should be considered for referral to a haematologist for investigation (e.g. prothrombotic screen and bone marrow examination).

• Cross-sectional radiological imaging may have been performed to establish the diagnosis; if not, it may be indicated if intra-abdominal malignancy or infection is suspected as a cause.

What are the management options?

Treatment varies depending upon the time course of presentation and the severity of the hepatocellular dysfunction:

• *Fulminant hepatic failure*: Urgent liver transplantation may be required.

• *Acute or chronic presentation*: Ascites may be managed with diuretics although up to half of cases are diuretic resistant from the outset. In selected cases, insertion of a transjugular intrahepatic portosystemic shunt (TIPS) can be useful providing it is possible to gain access to the obstructed hepatic venous system. If these options are unsuccessful or not possible, liver transplantation may be required. Patients should be considered for anticoagulant therapy.

Hepatic venography was performed which demonstrated complete obstruction in the hepatic veins. Careful cannulation of the right hepatic vein revealed an elevated venous pressure with sluggish blood flow. The obstruction was dilated by inflating a balloon, with improvement in blood flow and reduction in venous pressure. Next the middle hepatic vein was cannulated and a balloon inflated, resulting in improved venous flow and a reduction in the venous pressure gradient (Fig. 10.2). It was not possible to cannulate the left hepatic vein. During the procedure a transjugular liver biopsy was obtained that demonstrated centrilobular congestion.

Following the procedure her ascites rapidly improved and her liver function tests returned to normal. She was referred to a haematologist for further investigation. Bone marrow examination was normal with no evidence of a myeloproliferative disorder. Her procoagulant screen revealed that she has factor V Leiden mutation.

What is factor V Leiden mutation?

Factor V is a protein of the blood coagulation cascade. The factor V Leiden mutation results in a single amino acid change and makes factor V resistant to cleavage by activated protein C. Factor V therefore remains active and increases the rate of thrombin generation resulting in hypercoagulability. Factor V Leiden is the commonest hereditary prothrombotic disorder. Heterozygotes are affected and may present with venous thrombosis, particularly deep vein thrombosis or pulmonary embolus. Homozygotes have a more severe clinical condition.

She is started on lifelong warfarin anticoagulation and advised to stop smoking and to cease the oral contraceptive pill.

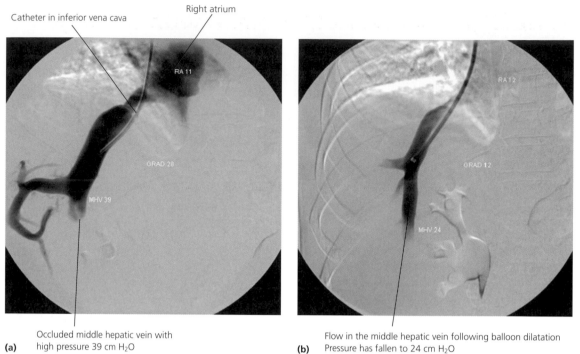

Catheter in inferior vena cava

Right atrium

Occluded middle hepatic vein with
high pressure 39 cm H_2O

(a)

Flow in the middle hepatic vein following balloon dilatation
Pressure has fallen to 24 cm H_2O

(b)

Figure 10.2 Hepatic venography before (a) and after (b) balloon dilatation of the occluded middle hepatic vein in this patient.

CASE REVIEW

This young woman presented acutely with the triad of abdominal pain, ascites and hepatomegaly. Ultrasound investigation demonstrated obstruction to hepatic venous flow which was confirmed on venography. She was treated by dilating two of her hepatic veins, which successfully decompressed her liver resulting in disappearance of the ascites. She had several risk factors for developing venous thrombosis: she was a smoker, she took the oral contraceptive pill and she had a positive family history. Investigation revealed that she had the factor V Leiden mutation and she was therefore started on long-term anticoagulation.

KEY POINTS

- Hepatic venous outflow obstruction can be caused by occlusion of the hepatic venules, the main hepatic veins or the inferior vena cava
- The presentation may be acute (including fulminant liver failure) or chronic
- The main presenting features are abdominal pain, tender hepatomegaly and ascites
- Myeloproliferative disorders or prothrombotic tendencies are the commonest underlying causes of hepatic venous thrombosis
- Treatment options include simple management of ascites with diuretics, interventional radiological treatments to open the occluded veins and liver transplantation

Case 11 A 40-year-old woman with lethargy and pruritus

Maureen Wilcox, a 40-year-old solicitor presents to her GP with a progressive history of tiredness and pruritus. She has vitiligo and a past history of rheumatoid arthritis that is in remission.

What are the main differential diagnoses?

Tiredness is a very non-specific symptom that is associated with many disease processes, both physical and psychological. Pruritus may be due to a primary skin condition or a manifestation of a systemic illness. Causes include:

- Skin conditions (e.g. scabies, eczema, urticaria).
- Liver disease (cholestasis).
- Malignancy (e.g. lymphoma, some carcinomas).
- Haematological disease (e.g. polycythaemia rubra vera).
- Renal disease (chronic renal failure with uraemia).
- Metabolic disease (e.g. hyperthyroidism, carcinoid syndrome).
- Pregnancy.
- Miscellaneous (e.g. drugs, psychogenic).

Why do people with liver disease get pruritus?

The exact reason why people with liver disease get pruritus is unclear. It is often a feature of cholestatic liver disease, when the flow of bile is obstructed either at the intrahepatic or extrahepatic level. As a result of the inability of the liver to excrete bile, bile acids are retained in the blood and it is thought that this is what leads to itching. There is also a suggestion that liver disease leads to an increase in naturally occurring opioid agonists and these contribute to the itching.

Hepatology: Clinical Cases Uncovered, 1st edition. © Kathryn Nash and Indra Neil Guha. Published 2011 by Blackwell Publishing Ltd.

How would you approach this patient if you were the general practitioner?

Any patient presenting with generalised, non-specific symptoms requires a detailed history and examination to look for a physical cause for their symptoms. A series of blood tests are required to screen for serious underlying pathology such as systemic disease and malignancy:

- *Full blood count*: Anaemia may be associated with malignancy or renal failure. A haematological disorder or lymphoma may cause anaemia, polycythaemia or other changes in the full blood count.
- *Renal function*: Advanced renal failure may cause tiredness and lethargy and patients with uraemia may have pruritus.
- *Liver function tests*: Cholestatic liver disease is characteristically associated with an elevation in the alkaline phosphatase. Patients may have other abnormalities of liver function such as raised bilirubin and aminotransferases. Marked cholestasis can, however, occur in the absence of jaundice and patients may have a normal bilirubin.
- *Thyroid function tests*: Tiredness is a common feature of thyroid disorders. Pruritus can be a feature of hyperthyroidism or hypothyroidism.
- *Erythrocyte sedimentation rate (ESR)*: The ESR is a non-specific indicator of the presence of disease. If elevated it suggests a systemic inflammatory, infectious or malignant process.

Physical examination reveals a well looking woman with palmar erythema but no other signs of chronic liver disease. She has bilateral xanthelasma. Abdominal examination is normal. Her blood tests are normal apart from a raised alkaline phosphatase of 312 iU/L (normal 35–105 iU/L).

What are the causes of a raised alkaline phosphatase?

- *Liver disease*: Alkaline phosphatase (ALP) is present in the biliary canalicular membranes of the liver. Levels are raised in cholestasis of any cause, whether intrahepatic or extrahepatic disease. Raised levels may also occur in hepatic infiltration, e.g. metastatic cancer, and in cirrhosis. In hepatic inflammation levels may also be elevated but other liver function tests are also frequently abnormal, particularly aminotransferases (e.g. ALT).

• *Bone*: A different isoenzyme of ALP is produced by osteoblasts in the bone. It is elevated in Paget's disease, growing children, osteomalacia, metastases, hyperparathyroidism and renal failure.

• *Other*: The placenta secretes its own ALP isoenzyme, therefore raised levels can be seen in pregnancy. The cells lining the intestine and the proximal convoluted tubule of the kidney also produce ALP although it is rare for enzymes produced from these sites to account for an elevation in total ALP.

How could you confirm that the elevated ALP was due to a hepatic cause?

• Gamma glutamyl transferase (γ-GT) is a microsomal enzyme that is present in the liver. In cholestasis the γ-GT rises in parallel with the ALP as it has a similar pathway of excretion. Therefore a rise in both ALP and γ-GT is highly suggestive of liver disease. Drugs such as alcohol and phenytoin induce the activity of γ-GT, thus a mild elevation of γ-GT alone may be due to moderate alcohol intake and does not necessarily indicate liver disease.

• The isoenzymes of ALP can be differentiated by electrophoretic separation. In the absence of clinical signs or other laboratory abnormalities it is occasionally necessary to identify the source of an elevated ALP in this way.

Mrs Wilcox's γ-GT is elevated at 185 U/L (normal 11–50 U/L). Further questioning reveals that she does not consume any alcohol. She is referred to the hepatology clinic.

What key questions should be asked to help identify the cause of the cholestasis?

• *Pain*: The presence of pain would be suggestive of extrahepatic biliary obstruction, particularly that caused by gallstones.

• *Weight loss*: Weight loss may indicate a malignant process, e.g. malignant infiltration of the liver or obstruction by pancreatic or bile duct cancer (known as cholangiocarcinoma), but can also occur in the advanced stages of cirrhosis.

• *Drug history*: Many drugs can cause cholestatic hepatitis, therefore a full detailed drug history is mandatory. The history of drug exposure may predate the development of cholestasis by many weeks. Intrahepatic cholestasis is a common manifestation of drug-mediated hepatotoxicity and many drugs have been implicated, including:
   ○ Sex hormones, anabolic steroids.
   ○ Antibiotics, e.g. erythromycin, flucloxacillin, amoxicillin (particularly when given with clavulonic acid as co-amoxiclav), nitrofurantoin.
   ○ Azathioprine.
   ○ Chlorpromazine.

• *Associated disorders*: The presence of other autoimmune diseases would point towards an immune-mediated liver disease such as primary biliary cirrhosis or primary sclerosing cholangitis.

• *Pregnancy*: Obstetric cholestasis typically presents with pruritus. It usually occurs in the third trimester of pregnancy, ALP levels may be elevated due to placental or liver production. Serum bile acids are frequently elevated.

How would you narrow down the differential diagnosis?

A liver ultrasound is mandatory to determine the level of biliary obstruction. In extrahepatic biliary obstruction ultrasound typically demonstrates biliary duct dilatation. The absence of a dilated biliary system on liver ultrasound is suggestive of intrahepatic cholestasis.

Mrs Wilcox's hepatologist organised for her to have a liver ultrasound. This demonstrates that her liver is enlarged but with a normal echotexture. There is no biliary duct dilatation.

What further investigations would you do?

The absence of biliary duct dilatation suggests intrahepatic cholestasis (Box 11.1). A careful drug history must be taken to exclude drug-mediated cholestasis. Further investigations include:

• Chronic liver disease screen.
• Liver autoimmune profile and immunoglobulins.
• Chronic viral screen, particularly hepatitis B and C.
• Metabolic screen (ferritin, caeruloplasmin, α_1-antitrypsin level).
• Consideration for liver biopsy (may not be necessary if the diagnosis is clear from the history and chronic liver

> **Box 11.1 Causes of intrahepatic cholestasis**
>
> - Primary biliary cirrhosis
> - Primary sclerosing cholangitis
> - Drugs
> - Obstetric cholestasis
> - Viral infection (some hepatitis viruses cause a predominantly cholestatic injury, e.g. hepatitis E)
> - Benign recurrent intrahepatic cholestasis (a rare familial disorder with recurrent episodes of jaundice with pruritus, often beginning in childhood. Patients are well in between episodes. Progression to chronic liver disease is rare)

> **Box 11.2 Features of PBC**
>
> - Female to male ratio is 9 : 1
> - Age of presentation is typically 40–50 years
> - Most frequent in Europe and North America where the prevalence is c. 50 per 10^6 population
> - Unknown aetiology, possible aberrant immunological response to an unknown microorganism
> - Presence of antimitochondrial antibody (M2) in c. 95%

disease screen or if there is a clear drug history and the patient improves on cessation of the drug).

What is the most likely diagnosis?

This woman has symptoms of lethargy and pruritus, intrahepatic cholestasis and a past history of autoimmune disease. This is suggestive of an autoimmune cholestatic liver disease. The most likely diagnosis is primary biliary cirrhosis.

What is primary biliary cirrhosis?

Primary biliary cirrhosis (PBC) is a chronic disorder in which there is progressive destruction of the bile ducts. The aetiology is unknown but immunological mechanisms may play a part. Patients typically present with symptoms of fatigue and pruritus. The natural history of PBC is variable but the majority of symptomatic patients develop progressive liver disease eventually leading to cirrhosis (Box 11.2).

What laboratory abnormalities are characteristic of PBC?

- *Raised alkaline phosphatase*: High serum ALP is often the only abnormality in the liver biochemistry. Patients on treatment frequently have completely normal liver function tests.
- *Mitochondrial antibodies*: Antibodies to mitochondria (AMA) are present in over 95% of patients. The M2 antibody is specific to PBC; a positive AMA screening test must therefore be followed up with testing for the M2 subtype to prevent false positive results. The presence of AMA in high titre is unrelated to the clinical or histological picture and may play no part in its pathogenesis. Up

to 5% of cases have identical biochemical and histological features without AMA and are termed AMA-negative PBC.
- *Raised serum cholesterol*: Cholesterol metabolism is markedly deranged in patients with PBC leading to hypercholesterolaemia, which can be severe. Signs such as xanthoma and xanthelasma may be present. Most studies suggest that there is no increased risk of ischaemic heart disease in patients with PBC and hypercholesterolaemia and it remains uncertain whether the hyperlipidaemia of PBC should be treated.
- *Raised serum IgM*: There is an increased synthesis of IgM, thought to be due to a failure of the switch from IgM to IgG during antibody synthesis.
- *Raised bilirubin*: Jaundice is a late feature of PBC and patients should be considered for liver transplantation when this develops.

What disorders are associated with PBC?

- *Autoimmune disease*: Other autoimmune diseases are frequently seen in patients with PBC, e.g. rheumatoid arthritis, Sjögren's syndrome, thyroid disorders, scleroderma and coeliac disease.
- *Bone disease*: Bone disease is common in patients with PBC:
  - *Osteopaenia and osteoporosis*: female sex, malabsorption and a possible direct inhibitory effect of bilirubin on osteoblasts contribute to osteopaenia.
  - *Osteomalacia*: cholestasis may result in malabsorption of fat-soluble vitamins leading to vitamin D deficiency. Furthermore, sequestration of vitamin D in the gut by drugs used to treat PBC, such as cholestyramine, may contribute.
- *Others*: An association with disorders such as fibrosing alveolitis, renal tubular acidosis and membranous glomerulonephritis has been reported.

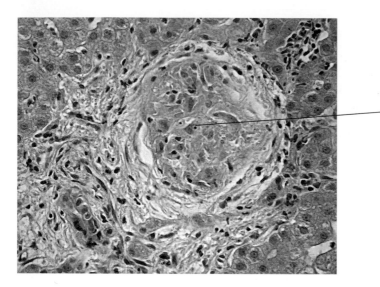

X

Figure 11.1 Liver biopsy taken from Mrs Wilcox demonstrating features of PBC.

Her antimitochondrial antibody is negative. Her hepatologist suspects that she has PBC based on her history but in the absence of a positive AMA recommends that she has a liver biopsy. This demonstrates classic features of primary biliary cirrhosis including necrotic bile ducts surrounded with early fibrosis (Fig. 11.1).

What feature is shown by X in Fig. 11.1? What is it composed of? What other causes of this liver biopsy feature do you know?

Figure 11.1 illustrates a hepatic granuloma. This is a collection of immune cells, principally macrophages, which form in response to an injury that the body cannot eliminate (e.g. chronic infection, chronic inflammation). The macrophages can fuse to form multinucleate giant cells. Granulomas may contain necrotic material in their centre, when they are known as caseating granulomas, a feature typically seen in granulomas associated with tuberculosis. In PBC the granulomas are normally concentrated around the portal tracts. Other causes of granulomas on liver biopsy are given in Box 11.3.

After making a diagnosis of PBC what would you tell the patient?

It is important to inform her that in most cases PBC is a gradually progressive disorder. She therefore needs to regularly attend the outpatient clinic to monitor her condition and to screen for treatable complications, e.g. oesophageal varices and osteoporosis.

Box 11.3 Causes of granulomas on liver biopsy

- PBC (granulomas typically around the bile ducts)
- Sarcoidosis (granulomas thoughout the liver parenchyma)
- Lymphoma, Hodgkin's disease
- Infection
  - bacterial, e.g. tuberculosis, brucellosis
  - parasitic, e.g. schistosomiasis, strongyloides
  - viral, e.g. HIV, HCV
  - fungal, e.g. histoplasmosis, coccidiomycosis
- Drug hypersensitivity (e.g. phenylbutazone, sulphonamide)
- Erythema nodosum
- Foreign body (e.g. talc, suture)

The rate of progression of the disease is highly variable. Patients who are asymptomatic at presentation usually develop symptoms over 5–10 years. Once symptoms develop, the median time to progress to liver failure requiring transplantation is 10 years.

How should she be managed?

- *Lethargy*: The lethargy associated with PBC may be disabling. It is important to exclude coexisting treatable causes of lethargy including depression, anaemia, thyroid or adrenal disease. Otherwise the patient should be given symptomatic advice.

- *Pruritus*:
  ◦ *Cholestyramine*: this non-absorbable anion exchange resin binds bile acids in the intestine and prevents their reabsorption in the ileum and is the first-line treatment for pruritus in PBC. It is effective in up to 90% of patients but is unpleasant to ingest and causes constipation.
  ◦ *Ursodeoxycholic acid*: this is an endogenous bile acid that can improve the itch associated with PBC. It has also been shown to improve liver function tests and slow progression of liver disease. Some studies suggest that it might delay the need for liver transplantation. Most patients are therefore given ursodeoxycholic acid for its role in treating PBC itself.
  ◦ *Antihistamines*: these drugs are usually given at night and the main benefit is probably related to their sedative effect.
  ◦ *Rifampicin*: the antibiotic rifampicin has been shown to be effective in treating cholestasis-associated pruritus although its mechanism of action is unknown.
  ◦ *Opioid receptor antagonists*: in patients who do not respond to the above medications the orally active opioid receptor antagonist naltrexone may be beneficial.
  ◦ *Liver transplantation*: rarely patients are refractory to treatment and so disabled by pruritus that liver transplantation is considered for this symptom.
- *Bone disease*: Vitamin D deficiency should be sought and replacement given if found to be deficient. Patients should have regular DEXA (dual energy X-ray absorptiometry) bone densitometry and be given calcium supplements or bisphosphonates if appropriate.

Mrs Wilcox is started on cholestyramine and ursodeoxycholic acid which control her symptoms and she defaults from regular clinic follow-up. Eight years later she re-presents with jaundice, ascites and a bilirubin of 150 μmol/L.

What management steps would you consider now?

Whilst it is most likely that her deterioration is due to the gradual progression of PBC, it is important to exclude other precipitants for her symptoms:

- *Exclude hepatocellular carcinoma*: Patients with advanced PBC are at risk of hepatocellular carcinoma, therefore she should undergo radiological imaging (e.g. ultrasound) to exclude the development of a tumour as a cause of her deterioration.
- *Exclude a vascular problem*: Patients with cirrhosis may develop a disturbance in portal venous flow due to the increased stiffness of the liver. Development of portal vein thrombosis can cause deterioration in liver function and should be sought by ultrasound with Doppler or CT/MRI imaging with portal phase contrast.
- *Exclude an additional liver disease*: Patients with chronic liver disease who deteriorate should always be evaluated for the possibility of a superadded liver disease. Investigations should be undertaken to exclude biliary obstruction such as that by gallstones (ultrasound), viral hepatitis or other autoimmune liver disease.
- *Exclude drug-toxicity*: Patients who deteriorate should always be asked about any drugs (prescribed or over the counter remedies) that could have caused liver injury and precipitated deterioration.
- *Consider for liver transplantation*: If there is no precipitant for her deterioration identified then she should be considered for liver transplantation (Box 11.4).

Mrs Wilcox is assessed and placed on the waiting list for liver transplantation and a suitable donor is found 8 months later. The transplant is uncomplicated and she is alive and well 3 years later.

Box 11.4 Indications for liver transplantation in PBC

- Increasing jaundice (generally consider when bilirubin is approaching 100 μmol/L)
- Intractable ascites
- Spontaneous bacterial peritonitis
- Encephalopathy
- Early hepatocellular carcinoma
- Unacceptable quality of life (e.g. intractable pruritus)

CASE REVIEW

This woman had a history of autoimmune diseases and presented with classic features of primary biliary cirrhosis (lethargy, pruritus and a raised alkaline phosphatase). Ninetyfive percent of patients with PBC have a positive M2 antimitochondrial antibody and this, along with a typical history and biochemical picture, is usually sufficient to make the diagnosis. In this case, AMA was negative; there-fore she underwent a liver biopsy, which demonstrated granulomatous destruction of the bile ducts confirming the diagnosis of AMA-negative PBC. She was treated with cholestyramine and ursodeoxycholic acid, which control-led her symptoms, but her liver disease progressed and she required liver transplantation.

KEY POINTS

- Lethargy and pruritus are non-specific symptoms that require investigation as they may have a serious cause
- A raised alkaline phosphatase can indicate liver or bone disease and may be seen in pregnancy
- Primary biliary cirrhosis is an autoimmune disorder of the liver leading to progressive damage of the intrahepatic bile ducts leading to cholestasis and progression to cirrhosis
- If a patient has typical symptoms, biochemistry and a positive M2 antimitochondrial antibody, liver biopsy may not be required to make the diagnosis
- Treatment is aimed at controlling symptoms:
  - lethargy – exclude other causes
  - pruritus – cholestyramine, ursodeoxycholic acid, antihistamines, rifampicin, naltrexone
  - bone disease – vitamin D, calcium, bisphosphonates
- Ursodeoxycholic acid may improve liver biochemistry and slow progression of liver disease
- Liver transplantation remains the only effective treatment for patients with end-stage disease

A 25-year-old woman with malaise and elevated liver enzymes

Ann Jones, a 25-year-old finance director consults her general practitioner because she has been feeling increasingly tired over the past 6 months. There are no other symptoms and physical examination is unremarkable. She has type 1 diabetes and receives regular insulin. She also suffers from hypothyroidism for which she receives thyroxine treatment. She is on no other medication. The GP arranges some blood investigations that reveal that her ALT is elevated at 287 iU/L.

What should you do next?

• There are many causes of tiredness. In this particular case it is important to ensure that her other chronic conditions are under control by checking her thyroid function tests and reviewing her diabetic control as well as performing additional screening bloods including a full blood count, urea and electrolytes and erythrocyte sedimentation rate (ESR).

• An elevated ALT should prompt further investigation to look for causes of hepatitis:
  ○ Viral hepatitis serology
  ○ Immunoglobulins and liver autoautibodies
  ○ Ferritin
  ○ Caeruloplasmin
  ○ Alpha-1 antitrypsin level.

• A liver ultrasound should be performed which may reveal information about liver size, shape and texture (bright suggesting fat infiltration, coarse suggesting fibrosis) and whether there is any focal pathology. A normal liver ultrasound does not exclude significant hepatology pathology however.

• The liver function tests should be repeated and if the abnormality persists the patient should be referred for further investigation.

Her full blood count, urea and electrolytes and thyroid function tests are normal. HbA1C is satisfactory at 6.2%. Repeat liver function tests are as follows:

Bilirubin	13 μmol/L
ALT	301 iU/L
ALP	102 iU/L
Albumin	35 g/L

Further blood results reveal that viral hepatitis serology is negative, and that caeruloplasmin, α_1-antitrypsin and ferritin levels are normal. Her immunoglobulins are significantly elevated with an IgG of 35 g/L (normal 6–16 g/L). The autoantibody screen is as follows:

Antinuclear antibody	Positive
Anti-smooth muscle antibody	Positive
Liver kidney microsomal antibody	Negative
Antimitochondrial antibody	Negative

What are the causes of elevated immunoglobulins?

• *Polyclonal increase*:
  ○ Chronic infection, e.g. HIV, parasite infection
  ○ Chronic autoimmune disease, e.g. autoimmune hepatitis
  ○ Chronic inflammation, e.g. cirrhosis, sarcoidosis.
• *Monoclonal increase*:
  ○ Multiple myeloma
  ○ Monoclonal gammopathy of unknown significance
  ○ Lymphoma
  ○ Waldenström's macroglobuminaemia.

What is the most likely diagnosis?
Autoimmune hepatitis.

What are the characteristics of this condition?
As with other autoimmune disorders, autoimmune hepatitis occurs more frequently in young and middle-aged women. Patients may present in several ways:

Hepatology: Clinical Cases Uncovered, 1st edition. © Kathryn Nash and Indra Neil Guha. Published 2011 by Blackwell Publishing Ltd.

• *Chronic hepatitis*: Most patients present with non-specific symptoms such as tiredness and right upper quadrant pain or are detected incidentally following investigation for raised transaminases. Clinical examination may reveal signs of chronic liver disease, e.g. palmar erythema, spider naevi and hepatosplenomegaly.

• *Cirrhosis*: As chronic autoimmune hepatitis is often asymptomatic up to 25% of patients may have cirrhosis at presentation.

• *Acute hepatitis*: Up to 25% present with an acute hepatitis and may have jaundice.

• *Liver failure*: Rarely patients present with fulminant liver failure and liver transplantation is necessary if clinically appropriate.

In the majority of cases there are positive autoantibodies against nuclei (antinuclear antibodies), smooth muscle actin and occasionally mitochondria. Younger people may have positive liver kidney microsomal antibodies which define a more aggressive illness.

What conditions are associated with autoimmune hepatitis?

• Other autoimmune conditions, e.g. autoimmune thyroid disease, haemolysis, vitiligo, rheumatoid arthritis, inflammatory bowel disease, etc.

• Overlap syndromes are conditions with features similar to autoimmune hepatitis but with markers or symptoms to suggest other autoimmune liver disease. For example antimitochondrial antibody positivity may suggest overlap with primary biliary cirrhosis, or biopsy features of biliary tract inflammation may occur in overlap with primary sclerosing cholangitis.

• Some drugs can cause a chronic hepatitis clinically, immunologically and histologically identical to autoimmune hepatitis (e.g. methyldopa, nitrofurantoin, isoniazid). Patients are often female and have positive liver autoantibodies. Improvement may follow drug withdrawal but relapse occurs if the drug is reintroduced.

> Her hepatologist requests a liver biopsy which demonstrates a portal infiltrate of lymphocytes and plasma cells with periportal hepatitis characteristic of autoimmune hepatitis. There is minimal fibrosis but no cirrhosis.

How is autoimmune hepatitis treated?

• *Prednisolone*: Corticosteroids are given with the aim of controlling the liver inflammation. Oral prednisolone is usually very effective but needs to be given long

Table 12.1 Side effects of steroid and azathioprine therapy.

Prednisolone	Azathioprine
Cosmetic (acne, moon-shaped face, dorsal hump, striae)	Nausea and vomiting
Weight gain	Rash
Osteoporosis	Arthralgia and myalgia
Hypertension	Leukopaenia
Diabetes mellitus	Hepatotoxicity
Cataracts	Teratogenicity?
Psychiatric symptoms (depression, psychosis)	Oncogenicity?
Increased infection	
Poor healing	
Adrenal suppression	

term when it is associated with serious side effects (Table 12.1).

• *Steroid-sparing agent (e.g. azathioprine)*: Immunosuppressive agents with fewer side effects than corticosteroids are given for maintenance therapy. Azathioprine is usually given in the first instance; it takes a few weeks to be effective so the steroid dose should not be reduced rapidly. Many patients require a combination of low dose prednisolone (5–10 mg/day) and azathioprine to control disease activity. Some patients are unable to tolerate azathioprine in which case alternative agents may be used such as 6-mercaptopurine or mycophenolate mofetil.

> Mrs Jones is started on oral prednisolone 30 mg a day. After 2 weeks of treatment her ALT has fallen to 18 iU/L. Azathioprine is gradually introduced over the next month and her steroids are cautiously reduced. After 6 months she is on maintenance treatment with azathioprine (1 mg/kg body weight) and 7.5 mg a day of prednisolone. Her ALT is normal and she feels well.

What else should be done?

She is on long-term corticosteroids, which puts her at significant risk of developing osteoporosis. Bone mineral density should be measured using dual energy X-ray absorptiometry (DEXA) to assess fracture risk. If she is at risk, bone protective medication should be prescribed. General measure such as good nutrition, including adequate dietary calcium intake, and physical activity should be encouraged.

What is her prognosis?

Providing she can maintain a remission her prognosis is very good as she does not yet have cirrhosis. In some cases, drug therapy can be withdrawn over a 1–2-year period and patients remain in remission; however, many cases relapse once therapy is withdrawn. Histological remission tends to lag behind clinical remission, therefore a follow-up biopsy 1–2 years after initiating therapy is often required to guide treatment withdrawal. Many patients require long-term azathioprine to maintain remission and some are dependent on a low dose of steroids as well. A few cases (<10%) develop progressive disease despite immunosuppression and require liver transplantation.

Over the course of the next year her steroids are reduced to 5mg a day. Her diabetes is proving hard to control and her hepatologist is keen to withdraw steroids if possible. A follow-up liver biopsy is performed that shows no inflammatory activity and only minimal fibrosis. Following this her prednisolone is withdrawn and she remains well on azathioprine monotherapy.

CASE REVIEW

This 25-year-old woman with a history of autoimmune disease (diabetes and thyroid) presented with non-specific symptoms and an elevated ALT. Autoimmune hepatitis was suspected from her elevated immunoglobulins and positive autoantibodies and this was confirmed on liver biopsy. She was started on immunosuppressive treatment with steroids and azathioprine which produced a biochemical remission. Liver biopsy 18 months later showed histological remission and her steroids were safely withdrawn.

KEY POINTS

- Presenting symptoms of autoimmune hepatitis are frequently non-specific
- Autoimmune hepatitis may progress to cirrhosis without any symptoms
- Acute presentation with jaundice and even liver failure can occur
- Autoimmune hepatitis is suggested by raised immunoglobulins and positive autoantibodies

- Treatment is with steroids initially to control inflammation and then the addition of a steroid-sparing agent to minimise the side effects of long-term steroid use
- Many patients require long-term treatment to maintain remission

PART 2: CASES

Case 13 Deranged liver function tests in a patient with ulcerative colitis

Mr Arthur Davies is a 42-year-old farmer who presents to his GP with fatigue and vague abdominal discomfort. He has a past medical history of ulcerative colitis which is maintained in remission by oral sulfasalazine preparations. Eight months ago Mr Davies underwent a laparoscopic cholecystectomy. His GP performs some blood tests:

Bilirubin	15 µmol/L
ALT	154 iU/L
ALP	987 iU/L
Albumin	38 g/L
γ-GT	787 U/L

What diagnoses should you consider?

• Retained stones in the common bile duct. The fact that this man has had a cholecystectomy does not preclude the diagnosis of gallstones. If the common bile duct was not explored (either by ERCP or during the operation) it may still contain gallstones. Alternatively they may have formed *de novo* within the liver and migrated to the common bile duct.
• Primary sclerosing cholangitis (PSC).
• Primary biliary cirrhosis (see Case 12).
• Secondary biliary cirrhosis can occur secondary to chronic obstruction of the biliary system either from stones or more commonly a biliary stricture. In the Far East liver flukes are another cause of secondary cirrhosis.
• Cholangiocarcinoma.
• Intrahepatic cholestasis: Causes include drug reactions and infiltrative conditions (e.g. metastatic carcinoma and lymphoma).

An ultrasound is organised for Mr Davies and this shows no evidence of duct dilatation or gallstones. A MRCP reveals an irregular biliary tree with beading but no dominant strictures (Fig. 13.1).

Hepatology: Clinical Cases Uncovered, 1st edition. © Kathryn Nash and Indra Neil Guha. Published 2011 by Blackwell Publishing Ltd.

What is the most likely diagnosis?

Primary sclerosing cholangitis (Box 13.1).

Mr Davies was commenced on ursodeoxycholic acid. In view of his pan-ulcerative colitis and diagnosis of PSC he was put on an annual colonoscopy surveillance programme. A bone scan showed he had early osteoporosis and he was commenced on calcium, vitamin D supplements and bisphosphonates. He was reviewed regularly in the hepatology outpatients and was symptomatically well with some improvement in his liver function tests.

Two years later he presents to his GP with pain, fevers and jaundice. Liver blood tests are shown below:

Bilirubin	78 µmol/l
ALT	87 iU/L
ALP	1209 iU/L
γ-GT	970 U/L

An ultrasound showed dilated intrahepatic ducts and no gallstones in the gallbladder.

What is the likely cause for the deterioration?

The most likely diagnosis is ascending cholangitis either due to: (i) dominant stricture related to PSC; or (ii) cholangiocarcinoma on the background of PSC.

Mr Davies is admitted to hospital for intravenous rehydration and analgesia, and antibiotics with ciprofloxacin are commenced.

What other tests should be organised?

• Tumour markers can be difficult to interpret in this setting as they are elevated in cholangitis and obstructive jaundice from benign or malignant causes. Extremely elevated levels of CA19.9 can be suggestive of a cholangiocarcinoma but are not diagnostic.
• Cross-sectional imaging should be organised, e.g. a CT scan.

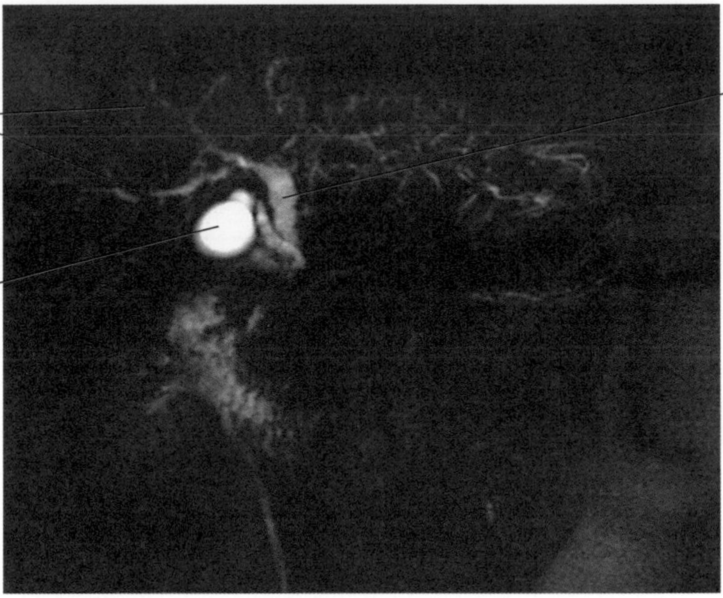

Intrahepatic ducts demonstrating irregularity due to stricturing

Irregular common hepatic duct

Gallbladder

Figure 13.1 MRCP demonstrating features of primary sclerosing cholangitis in this patient.

Box 13.1 Primary sclerosing cholangitis

- Strong male preponderance (70%)
- Exact pathophysiology is undetermined but there is evidence for a multifactorial aetiology including a genetic predisposition
- Strong association with inflammatory bowel disease:
  ○ approximately 70% of patients with PSC with have associated inflammatory bowel disease (in particular ulcerative colitis)
  ○ approximately 10% of patients with ulcerative colitis will have PSC
- The presentation of PSC can include symptoms of fatigue, right-sided abdominal pain, jaundice, fevers and weight loss

- Blood tests will typically show a cholestatic pattern with elevation in bilirubin, ALP and γ-GT. Autoantibodies may be positive but do not have a high sensitivity or specificity
- Diagnosis can be confirmed by MRCP or ERCP (Fig. 13.2), which may reveal strictures or 'beading' of the biliary tree
- In a minority of cases the cholangiogram is normal despite clinical and biochemical features suggestive of PSC. A liver biopsy in these cases will aid diagnosis by revealing periductal fibrosis and 'onion skin' appearance (Fig. 13.3)
- Treatment includes the use of ursodeoxycholic acid, but the only definitive treatment is orthotopic liver transplantation for those with decompensating liver disease

---

A CT scan shows no evidence of a mass lesion but confirms the presence of dilated intrahepatic ducts. An ERCP demonstrates the presence of a stricture in the common bile duct (Fig. 13.4). Brushings are taken from the stricture at ERCP and a plastic stent is inserted to allow drainage and relieve the obstruction. The brushings are sent for cytological examination which suggests high grade malignancy and a provisional diagnosis of cholangiocarcinoma is made (Box 13.2).

What are the treatment options?

• Depending on the anatomical location of the tumour, associated co-morbidity of the patient, extent of the liver disease and absence of metastatic spread, surgical resection is the preferred option.

• Palliative chemotherapy may increase life expectancy in carefully selected patients.

• Photodynamic therapy is an emerging treatment and involves the injection of a photosensitising agent. This is

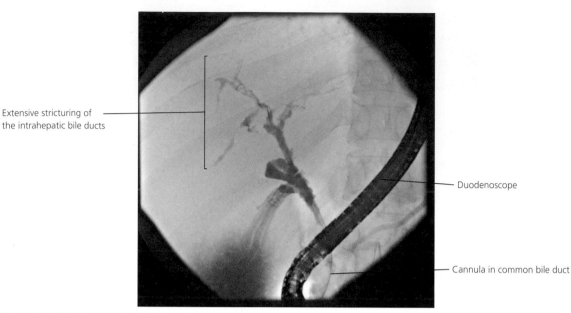

Extensive stricturing of the intrahepatic bile ducts

Duodenoscope

Cannula in common bile duct

Figure 13.2 ERCP demonstrating bile duct stricturing in PSC.

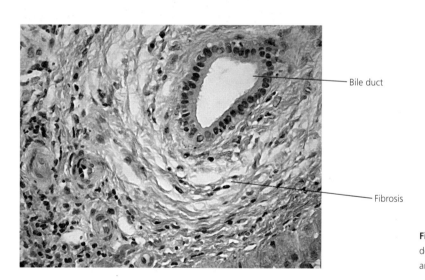

Bile duct

Fibrosis

Figure 13.3 Liver biopsy in PSC demonstrating 'onion skin' fibrosis around a bile duct.

retained by tumour cells for longer than normal tissue. When exposed to a certain frequency of light, administered at ERCP 24–48 hours following injection, it results in cell death. Further evidence is required to determine its efficacy and safety.

• Many cases are treated with palliative stenting of the biliary stricture.

• In most centres the presence of cholangiocarcinoma is a contraindication for orthotopic liver transplantation because of the high rate of recurrence.

Mr Davies has a surgical resection of his cholangiocarcinoma and makes a good recovery. He is discharged home and continues to be under careful follow-up 3 years later.

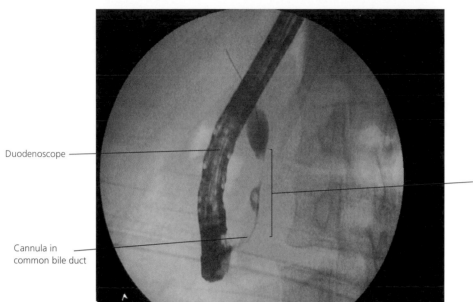

Duodenoscope

Malignant stricture of
the common bile duct

Cannula in
common bile duct

Figure 13.4 ERCP demonstrating common bile duct cholangiocarcinoma in this patient.

Box 13.2 Cholangiocarcinoma

- Adenocarcinoma arising from biliary epithelium
- May be intrahepatic or extrahepatic in origin. Further classification is made depending on the anatomical location of the tumour
- Reported to occur in up to 20% of patients with PSC. Other risk factors include:
  ○ smoking
  ○ history of inflammatory bowel disease
  ○ alcohol consumption
  ○ concomitant diagnosis of a colorectal tumour
- Symptoms can be non-specific but include weight loss, abdominal pain, increasing jaundice and ascending cholangitis

CASE REVIEW

A 42-year-old man with known ulcerative colitis presented with deranged liver function tests of an obstructive pattern. Subsequent imaging, using MRCP, revealed primary sclerosing cholangitis. Two years later he presented with cholangitis from a dominant stricture in the common bile duct. A cholangiocarcinoma was confirmed by brushings taken at ERCP. He had a liver resection following which he was alive and well with no recurrence 3 years later.

KEY POINTS

- There is an association between inflammatory bowel disease and primary sclerosing cholangitis
- A previous cholecystectomy should not exclude gallstones as a differential for obstructive jaundice
- The diagnosis of PSC can be made by MRCP, ERCP or liver biopsy
- The presence of PSC is a risk factor of the development of cholangiocarcinoma
- Patients with PSC and inflammatory bowel disease are also at increased risk of developing bowel cancer
- The treatment options for cholangiocarcinoma are limited but include surgical resection

PART 2: CASES

Case 14   Fatigue and deranged liver function tests in a patient with haemophilia

Mr Andrew Taylor is a 33-year-old with haemophilia who presents to his GP with fatigue. He has received factor 8 infusions for most of his life. His GP requests some standard tests and they return as below:

Bilirubin	15 μmol/L
ALT	74 iU/L
Albumin	38 g/L
Hb	13.9 g/dL
WBC	4.6 × 10⁹/L
Plt	176 × 10⁹/L
Thyroid function	Normal
EBV serology	IgM negative, IgG positive
CMV serology	Negative

How would you interpret these results and what further investigations would you request?

• He has positive serology for EBV but this suggests that he has had prior exposure rather than current infection (IgM negative and IgG positive). A PCR for EBV would clarify the diagnosis if there was any doubt.

• There is a mild transaminitis which needs investigation by a chronic liver disease screen.

The chronic liver disease screen returns with the following positive findings:

HCV IgG	Positive
PCR for HCV	900 000 iU/mL
Ultrasound	Normal appearance of liver, spleen and pancreas

What is the diagnosis?

Chronic hepatitis C virus (HCV) infection with active viral replication (Box 14.1).

Hepatology: Clinical Cases Uncovered, 1st edition. © Kathryn Nash and Indra Neil Guha. Published 2011 by Blackwell Publishing Ltd.

How did he acquire this infection?

Mr Taylor has received blood products for his haemophilia for many years. Prior to 1986, clotting factors derived from donated blood were frequently contaminated with viruses such as HCV. Nowadays the factor 8 is inactivated by heat or chemical treatment. Furthermore, recombinant factor 8 produced by genetic engineering is available and a proportion of patients are treated with this rather than factor 8 extracted from donated blood. Other risk factors for acquiring HCV are given in Box 14.2.

What are likely to be Mr Taylor's major concerns?

• Is he going to develop liver disease? As a haemophiliac he is highly likely to have known other people who have acquired chronic viral infections as a consequence of having received contaminated blood products. His major concern is probably going to be that he will develop liver failure or hepatocellular carcinoma.

• Is he at risk of passing the virus to others?

• Can he get rid of the virus?

What should you tell him about his diagnosis?

• He has chronic infection with HCV and has active viral replication.

• Patients chronically infected with HCV are highly unlikely to spontaneously clear the virus.

• About a third of people develop significant liver disease; risk factors exist that are associated with an increased likelihood of progression (Box 14.3).

• Treatments are available for HCV that can cure the virus in approximately 50% of cases.

• The virus can be passed on to others if there is blood exposure, e.g. sharing needles, but general household and sexual transmission is very low and no specific recommendations are made.

Box 14.1 HCV infection

- Acute illness is rarely symptomatic (<15% of cases)
- Most patients (c. 65–80%) with acute infection progress to chronic infection
- Chronic infection is often asymptomatic, therefore many people chronically infected are unaware that they carry the virus
- Blood tests will allow the distinction between prior exposure and clearance of virus (IgG positive and PCR negative) and current infection (IgG positive and PCR positive)
- The stage of liver disease is important to ascertain. Approximately 25% of patients with chronic hepatitis C will progress to cirrhosis

Box 14.2 Risk factors for acquiring HCV infection

- Intravenous drug abuse
- Blood products before 1991
- Tattooing or body piercing (particular if in unlicensed premises)
- Sexual transmission (risk is less than 1% but higher if there are multiple partners or history of traumatic intercourse)
- Haemodialysis
- Intranasal cocaine
- Needlestick injuries (less than 5%)
- Vertical transmission (less than 5%)

Box 14.3 Factors linked to accelerated progression of HCV-induced liver disease

- Male gender
- Older age at acquisition
- Alcohol
- Co-infection with HIV or chronic hepatitis B
- Obesity and insulin resistance

How do patients with HCV infection present?

- Acute hepatitis (rare; <15% of cases have a symptomatic illness).
- Often there are very few symptoms with chronic HCV but when present they can be non-specific and include tiredness, right upper quadrant pain, mood disturbance and rashes (including porphyria).

Box 14.4 Extrahepatic manifestations of HCV

- Eyes: retinopathy
- Skin: porphyria cutanea tarda, lichen planus, vasculitis (e.g. cryoglobuminaemia)
- Brain: cognition, depression, mood disturbance
- Kidney: vasculitis, glomerulonephritis
- Endocrine: thyroid dysfunction
- Rheumatology: arthritis, myalgia, Sjögren's syndrome
- Haematology: thrombocytopaenia, lymphoma

- HCV may be detected by a minor elevation in transaminases performed to investigate vague symptoms or found incidentally.
- Patients may present with decompensation of previously asymptomatic liver disease, e.g. jaundice, ascites, variceal haemorrhage.
- In addition to affecting the liver, HCV can also affect other organs (extrahepatic manifestations) and these are shown in Box 14.4.

What investigations should you do?
Assessment of the virus
- It is important to confirm that he is chronically infected and HCV RNA positive by repeating the test a few weeks later.
- Establishing which family of virus (genotype) is present will be helpful in advising him as to his chance of responding to treatment.

Assessment of the degree of liver disease
- Signs of significant liver dysfunction may include reduced albumin, prolonged clotting and low platelet count, raising the suspicion of underlying cirrhosis.
- Liver ultrasound to look for features of underlying cirrhosis.
- The present gold standard investigation for the staging of liver disease is histology obtained by a liver biopsy. In this a case a transabdominal approach may not be suitable, because of the bleeding diathesis associated with haemophilia, and therefore a transjugular approach may be more appropriate.
- Non-invasive tests for assessing fibrosis are an emerging area.

Other investigations
It is important to screen for other blood-borne viruses that he is also at risk of having acquired, e.g. HIV and hepatitis B virus.

What treatment is available?

• The standard care of treatment at the current time of writing is pegylated interferon (given as an injection once a week) and an oral tablet called ribavarin.

• Currently, treatment duration is 24–48 weeks depending on the genotype of virus, viral response to treatment and underlying liver disease severity.

• The response to treatment is dependent on a number of factors including the genotype of virus and severity of the underlying liver disease – those with severe fibrosis or cirrhosis are less likely to respond to therapy. Currently, the overall sustained viral response rate (undetectable virus by PCR 6 months after stopping treatment) is between 40% and 60% (over 80% in certain genotypes, e.g. genotype 2 and 3).

• There are common side effects of antiviral treatment (Box 14.5). The support of well-trained nurse specialists in viral hepatitis C to support, manage and educate patients is a cornerstone of managing patients with chronic viral hepatitis.

• Novel treatments for HCV are currently being tested in clinical trials.

Mr Taylor is found to have genotype 2 HCV. After a careful discussion with the patient he elects to have a transjugular liver biopsy. This reveals mild fibrosis, with no evidence of cirrhosis, and portal tract inflammation consistent with chronic hepatitis C. He is initiated on combination antiviral therapy with pegylated interferon and ribavarin for 6 months. He tolerates antiviral therapy well. His viral load initially declines but he does not achieve a sustained viral response 6 months after treatment (he still has virus detectable by PCR). Mr Taylor is kept under regular follow-up to monitor his condition and also to keep him informed about new clinical trials that are emerging for treating the virus. Unfortunately he stops attending the liver clinic and also stops seeing his GP. Six years later he presents to his GP with a distended abdomen and jaundice.

Box 14.5 Side effects of antiviral treatment

• Depression
• Flu-like symptoms
• Mood disturbance
• Anaemia
• Alopecia
• Thyroid disorders

What are the likely causes for his deterioration?

He is showing evidence of liver decompensation; the major differentials are:

• Progressive liver disease from his underlying chronic hepatitis C (Box 14.6). The development of cirrhosis in this man would be unusual (mild fibrosis to cirrhosis in 6 years) in the presence of hepatitis C virus alone. The other possibility is that he had more severe fibrosis at diagnosis but this was underscored because of sampling errors with the liver biopsy.

Box 14.6 Progression of liver disease in patients with chronic HCV infection

• Progression of liver fibrosis will vary between individual patients
• Approximately 25% of patients with chronic hepatitis C will develop cirrhosis
• The starting point of the liver fibrosis will obviously determine how long it takes to develop cirrhosis (e.g. if HCV is diagnosed in a patient with no fibrosis it can take 20–30 years to develop cirrhosis; if they have moderate fibrosis progression at diagnosis it may be much quicker)
• Fibrosis progression is not linear, and may accelerate with increasing disease severity (Fig. 14.1)

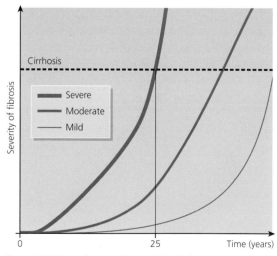

Figure 14.1 Rate of progression to cirrhosis depends upon the severity of fibrosis at initial biopsy.

- Accelerated liver disease from a second aetiological agent.
- The development of an underlying hepatocellular carcinoma (Box 14.7).
- The development of a portal vein thrombosis.

Upon further questioning Mr Taylor admits to having some major life events following antiviral treatment. His girlfriend left him shortly after his treatment stopped and he became very depressed. He started drinking vodka every night with a weekly intake of 70 units.

Mr Taylor is found to have ascites but there is no evidence of HCC or portal vein thrombosis. A transjugular liver biopsy shows advanced liver disease from a combination of alcohol and hepatitis C but no evidence of alcoholic hepatitis. He accepts counselling for his alcohol dependence. He is kept under very careful follow-up and commenced on diuretics. His synthetic function and ascites show limited improvement over the next 8 months. During this period the clinicians, alcohol liaison nurses and viral hepatitis nurses are confident that he has not returned to drinking excessively (random

alcohol levels have also been negative) and he is referred for orthotopic liver transplantation. He has careful assessment at the liver transplantation centre including psychological and psychiatric consultations before a decision upon transplantation is agreed. Twelve months later he has an orthotopic liver transplantation and makes an uneventful recovery.

What happens to hepatitis C following liver transplantation?

- Although HCV primarily infects the liver, small amounts of virus are present in extrahepatic sites and infection of the new liver is almost universal after transplantation.
- In the context of immunosuppression, the progression to cirrhosis is accelerated with 10–30% patients progressing to cirrhosis within 5 years of transplantation.
- Antiviral treatment can be difficult in this group for a number of reasons:
  ○ The treatment is less efficacious compared to the pretransplant setting.
  ○ Side effects of antiviral medication can be more common and severe in this group.
  ○ Antiviral therapy with agents such as interferon can potentially precipitate rejection of the graft.
- If significant liver damage develops in the graft, as assessed currently by liver biopsy, then treatment decisions are undertaken on an individual case basis and at specialist centres.

Box 14.7 Hepatocellular carcinoma and portal vein thrombosis

- Hepatocellular carcinoma (HCC) usually develops on the background of liver cirrhosis in HCV. Once liver cirrhosis is established the annual incidence of HCC has been reported to be approximately 5%
- The diagnosis of HCC should be actively excluded in patients who have a sudden decompensation (see Case 17). Once cirrhosis has been established it is important for patients to be part of a screening programme for HCC with 6-month to annual abdominal ultrasounds in combination with α-fetoprotein
- The treatment for HCC will depend on the size of the tumour, local invasion and the general health of the patient
- Portal vein thrombosis can occur in liver cirrhosis due to portal hypertension (it may also signify the development of an associated HCC). Doppler examination of the portal vein may reveal reversal of blood flow and cross-sectional imaging with triple phase will delineate the extent of thrombosis

What happens to haemophilia after liver transplantation?

Factor 8 is made in the liver. As the new liver does not have an error in factor 8 synthesis the patient is cured of haemophilia.

Mr Taylor was followed up regularly. HCV was detected in his blood but remained at a low level. Follow-up liver biopsies showed some mild inflammation, consistent with hepatitis C, but no significant fibrosis. Four years following his transplant he remains well. He is in a new relationship and is working full time as a computer analyst. He remains teetotal. He no longer requires any treatment for his haemophilia.

CASE REVIEW

A 23-year-old man with haemophilia presented with fatigue and abnormal liver function tests. Upon testing he was found to have chronic hepatitis C infection. He was genotype 1 and although he had antiviral therapy he was unable to clear the virus. Initial liver biopsy revealed mild fibrosis but 6 years later he presented with decompensated liver disease. During this time he admitted to drinking excessively and this contributed to the accelerated liver fibrosis. Despite abstinence, his synthetic liver function did not improve and he was considered for liver transplantation. He underwent successful liver transplantation and although he had some minor inflammation and recurrence of the virus, he was leading a normal life 4 years after transplantation.

KEY POINTS

- The symptoms of HCV can be non-specific, such as fatigue and mood disturbance, and in many cases there are no symptoms at all
- The majority of patients with acute infection develop chronic infection
- Testing directly for viraemia in the blood (PCR) will enable the diagnosis of active infection
- There are established treatments for chronic hepatitis C that are able to achieve a cure in over half of all cases
- Progression of liver fibrosis to cirrhosis will occur in approximately one-quarter of patients with HCV
- The time frame of fibrosis progression is variable but is accelerated by other aetiological agents such as alcohol
- Decompensated liver cirrhosis from hepatitis C is an indication for liver transplantation
- The recurrence of hepatitis C is common in the transplanted liver and is associated with accelerated liver fibrosis

Case 15 A 34-year-old man from Hong Kong with jaundice and vomiting

Tom Wong is a 34-year-old man originally from Hong Kong who has been living in the United Kingdom for the past 4 months. He presents to the emergency department with a short history of jaundice and vomiting. He is otherwise fit and well with no past medical history and he takes no regular medication. Direct questioning reveals that he has never used intravenous drugs and there is no history of recent foreign travel. He got married 5 months ago and his wife is his only sexual partner. Blood tests are as follows:

Bilirubin	127 μmol/L
ALT	947 iU/L
ALP	216 iU/L
INR	1.0
Hepatitis B surface antigen (HBsAg)	Positive
Hepatitis B surface antibody (anti-HBs)	Negative
Hepatitis B core IgM antibody (anti-HBc)	Positive

What is the diagnosis?

He has acute hepatitis B virus (HBV) infection based on the following evidence:
- He has hepatitis as evidenced by a raised alanine aminotransferase.
- He is positive for HBsAg and therefore has active HBV infection.
- IgM antibody to hepatitis B core (HBcAb) indicates an acute infection.

Important features of HBV are given in Box 15.1.

How common is HBV infection?

Worldwide, HBV infection is very common. It is estimated that over a billion people have been infected and that 400 million people remain chronic carriers of the virus. The prevalence of infection varies geographically:
- 0.1–2% in low prevalence areas (e.g. Western Europe, North America and Australasia).

> ### Box 15.1 Virology of hepatitis B virus
>
> - DNA virus belonging to the hepadnaviridae family of viruses
> - It has an outer envelope of virally encoded surface antigen (HBsAg), a viral core that encloses the viral polymerase and the viral genome – a circular, partially double-stranded DNA molecule (Fig. 15.1)
> - Different antigens are produced during infection and lead to a variety of antibody responses (see Table 15.2). Two proteins are produced from the area of the genome coding for the core protein: the core antigen itself (HBcAg) and the e antigen (HBeAg). They are produced from a single mRNA with HBeAg being initiated several nucleotides upstream from HBcAg. This produces a short signal peptide on HBeAg that allows it to be secreted into the blood whereas HBcAg, which lacks the signal peptide, is confined to the hepatocyte nucleus

- 3–5% in intermediate prevalence areas (e.g. Eastern Europe, Central Asia and South America).
- 10–20% in high prevalence areas (e.g. Southeast Asia and sub-Saharan Africa).

How is the virus transmitted from person to person?

HBV is spread parenterally, mainly via the blood or sexual transmission (Table 15.1).

What are the serological changes seen in acute hepatitis B infection with spontaneous recovery?

Following infection the first antigen detected is HBsAg (Table 15.2) – its detection precedes symptoms. Next HBeAg is detected and core antibodies (IgM and then IgG) are produced. HBeAg disappears from the serum accompanied by the development of anti-HBe. Finally, HBsAg disappears signifying viral clearance and anti-HBs is produced conferring long-term immunity.

Hepatology: Clinical Cases Uncovered, 1st edition. © Kathryn Nash and Indra Neil Guha. Published 2011 by Blackwell Publishing Ltd.

Table 15.1 Transmission of HBV.

Route of transmission	Notes
Vertical transmission (passage from mother to child at or shortly after birth)	Most common mode of transmission worldwide Now uncommon in developed countries due to antenatal screening and neonatal vaccination programmes
Sexual (heterosexual and male homosexual)	Important worldwide Dominant mode of transmission in developed countries
Blood borne	Intravenous drug use Transfusion of blood or blood products (uncommon in developed countries as blood is screened) Tattoos, acupuncture, body piercing
Close contact	Common mode of transmission between young children or among household contacts. HBV can survive outside the body for several days therefore transmission by contaminated toothbrushes, razors and even toys is possible

Table 15.2 Important serological tests for HBV infection.

Viral marker	Notes
Surface antigen (HBsAg)	First indication of viral infection Appears 1–10 weeks after exposure to the virus; may be detected before the onset of symptoms Most patients who recover from acute infection clear HBsAg within 4–6 months Persistence of HBsAg in serum for more than 6 months implies chronic infection
Surface antibody (anti-HBs)	Neutralising antibody that confers protective immunity against the virus Recovery from HBV infection occurs when HBsAg disappears and anti-HBs appears in the serum Also used to assess response to HBV vaccination
Core antigen (HBcAg)	HBcAg is an intracellular protein and is not detected in the blood
Core antibody (anti-HBc)	IgM anti-HBc is the first antibody produced following HBV infection IgM anti-HBc is the best screening test for acute HBV infection and may be the only antibody detectable during the window period between the disappearance of HBsAg and the detection of anti-HBs IgG anti-HBc is produced 2–4 months after infection and usually persists in the blood long term
e antigen (HBeAg)	HBeAg is produced from the same mRNA as HBcAg. It is initiated several nucleotides upstream producing a signal peptide that allows HBeAg to be secreted into the blood HBeAg-positive patients generally have high levels of HBV DNA in the serum and are highly infectious During acute infection, HBeAg is rapidly cleared and anti-HBe is produced In chronic infection HBeAg may persist for many years; seroconversion to anti-HBe usually occurs but it may be many decades after infection Loss of HBeAg is usually associated with the disappearance of HBV DNA from the serum and liver disease goes into remission. If this occurs before the patient develops cirrhosis the prognosis is generally very good
e antibody (anti-HBe)	Some anti-HBe-positive patients develop a mutation in the precore coding region and develop active viral replication (HBV DNA positivity) without detectable HBeAg in the blood. This 'precore mutant' virus may cause a particularly aggressive liver injury with rapid progression to cirrhosis

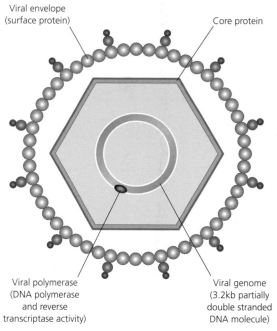

Figure 15.1 Hepatitis B virus particle.

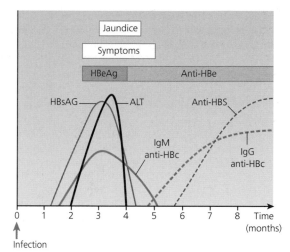

Figure 15.2 Serological changes in acute HBV infection.

The serological changes of acute HBV infection are shown in Fig. 15.2.

How may acute hepatitis B infection present clinically?

• *Subclinical infection or anicteric hepatitis*: In approximately 70% of patients infection is mild with either no symptoms at all or non-specific symptoms. The patient may clear the virus without knowing they have been exposed to it.

• *Icteric hepatitis*: A minority of patients develop a significant illness with jaundice (Box 15.2). Examination may reveal an enlarged tender liver and the spleen may be palpable. Transient rashes may occur and a few patients develop lymphadenopathy.

• *Fulminant hepatic failure*: Rarely (<0.5% of cases) acute hepatitis B infection results in massive hepatic necrosis and liver failure. This is characterised by coagulopathy, development of encephalopathy and death if liver transplantation is not undertaken.

• *Extrahepatic presentation*: Some patients present with extrahepatic manifestations of HBV infection, particularly immunological syndromes, e.g. rashes, polyarthritis, vasculitis or glomerulonephritis.

Box 15.2 Phases of illness in symptomatic acute HBV infection

• *Viral prodrome*: before the onset of hepatitis the patient is viraemic, which causes them to feel unwell with anorexia, nausea, headaches, malaise, abdominal discomfort and a low grade fever. Cigarette smokers may lose their taste for cigarettes

• *Hepatitis*: after 1–2 weeks the patient may develop jaundice, although not all patients become icteric. At the onset of jaundice the patient often feels better and the constitutional symptoms begin to resolve

• *Cholestasis*: the recovery phase is characterised by deepening jaundice associated with dark urine and pale stools due to the development of intrahepatic cholestasis. During this phase the patient may suffer from intense pruritus. Finally, the jaundice lessens and in the majority of cases symptoms resolve over 3–6 weeks

Tom feels unwell for a few days but he gradually improves and 2 weeks after presentation his jaundice has completely resolved. Blood tests taken 3 months after his initial presentation reveal:

Bilirubin	*14 μmol/L*
ALT	*42 iU/L*
ALP	*98 iU/L*
HBsAg	*Negative*
Anti-HBc IgG	*Positive*
Anti-HBs	*Positive*
Anti-HBc IgM	*Negative*

How do you interpret these blood tests?

• Hepatitis B surface antigen is negative therefore he has cleared the infection.
• Hepatitis B surface antibody is positive therefore he has produced a protective antibody to the virus.

What else should be done?

Hepatitis B infection is a notifiable illness and should be reported to the Health Protection Agency. It is important to try to ascertain how he acquired the virus and whether there is a risk that he could have passed it on to anyone else. It is important that his wife and family are screened for the presence of the virus.

Tom's wife, Amy, is also from Hong Kong. She is 10 weeks' pregnant and is in good health with no previous history of liver disease. She undergoes blood tests which reveal the following:

Bilirubin	13 μmol/L
ALT	27 iU/L
ALP	168 iU/L
Albumin	31 g/L
HBsAg	Positive
Anti-HBs	Negative
HBeAg	Positive
Anti-HBe	Negative
Anti-HBc IgM	Negative
Anti-HBc IgG	Positive
HBV DNA	Positive

How do you interpret her hepatitis B virus serology?

• The presence of HBsAg confirms that she is an active carrier of HBV.
• The absence of anti-HBc IgM antibody makes it very unlikely that this is an acute infection.

Is she infectious?

The antigen HBeAg is a marker of HBV replication and infectivity. She is HBeAg positive and has a high level of HBV DNA in the blood indicating that she is very infectious and at high risk of transmitting the virus to others. The most likely explanation for her husband's acute infection is that she has passed the virus on to him either sexually or via close household contact.

She has a high level of virus in her blood, why is she not unwell?

HBV itself is not directly cytopathic to hepatocytes. Liver damage only results in patients who produce a strong immune response to the virus when cytotoxic T lymphocytes cause lysis of infected hepatocytes. Amy is in the 'immunotolerant phase' of chronic hepatitis B infection characterised by active HBV replication in the liver, high levels of HBV DNA in the serum, but minimal immune response to the virus hence minimal liver damage. She is well with normal transaminases and if a liver biopsy were to be performed there would be no evidence of hepatocyte inflammation or necrosis.

In contrast, her husband developed an active immune response to the virus which is the explanation for him becoming unwell but also the reason why he cleared the virus whereas Amy has not. The T-lymphocyte response to the virus resulted in lysis of infected hepatocytes causing the rise in transaminases and, in his case, jaundice.

> **KEY POINT**
>
> • In hepatitis B virus infection, patients with a strong antiviral immune response are more likely to have a symptomatic illness but are more likely to clear the virus. The extreme example of this is fulminant liver failure when the immune response completely eradicates the virus but causes massive hepatic necrosis resulting in death unless the patient undergoes urgent transplantation

What is the explanation for her abnormal liver function tests?

She is pregnant. In pregnancy the alkaline phosphatase is frequently elevated as it is produced by the placenta. The albumin falls as a consequence of haemodilution due to the increased plasma volume characteristic of pregnancy.

How should her pregnancy be managed?

She is highly infectious and at risk of transmitting the virus to her baby at or around the time of birth. Infection acquired in the neonatal period is associated with a high risk of progression to chronic infection. As soon as the baby is born it should be given passive immunisation with hepatitis B immunoglobulin and receive a course of active immunisation in three doses at 0, 1 and 6 months.

Her pregnancy progresses uneventfully and her baby is given appropriate vaccination. Two years later her baby undergoes a blood test to see if he has responded to the vaccine. Results are as follows:

HBsAg	*Negative*
IgG anti-HBc	*Negative*
Anti-HBs	*Positive*

What do these results indicate?
• He is negative for HBsAg and is therefore not a chronic carrier of HBV.
• He is negative for IgG anti-HBc indicating that he did not acquire HBV infection.
• The presence of anti-HBs indicates that he has a protective immune response against the virus.

The HBV vaccine is a subunit vaccine, containing just HBsAg. As vaccine recipients are only exposed to this antigen they only produce anti-HBs, a neutralising antibody that effectively prevents infection. As they are not exposed to the whole virus, vaccine recipients will not produce anti-HBe or anti-HBc antibodies (Table 15.3).

Amy remains well in herself and defaults from regular clinical review. Five years later she is referred back to the hepatology service by her general practitioner who has found her to have abnormal liver function tests during routine testing. Blood tests reveal:

Bilirubin	*16 μmol/L*
ALT	*275 iU/L*
ALP	*154 iU/L*

What is the most likely explanation for her abnormal blood results?
She has probably moved from the immunotolerant phase into an immunoreactive phase. T lymphocytes are now recognising intracellular HBV antigens and causing lysis of infected hepatocytes. This leads to necroinflammation in the liver and the elevation in ALT. Most exacerbations of inflammation are asymptomatic, as in this case, but some are accompanied by symptoms of acute hepatitis.

This immunoreactive phase usually results in seroconversion from a HBeAg-positive to HBeAg-negative state with the development of anti-HBe (Fig. 15.3a). The ease with which she passes through this phase of HBeAg seroconversion is important in determining the extent of liver damage and her long-term prognosis. Some patients have a suboptimal immune response with recurrent exacerbations, repeated episodes of necroinflammation and have a high risk of developing cirrhosis.

What other possible explanations must be considered?
It is important to exclude other causes of liver disease and acute hepatitis by taking a full history. She should be asked about recent drug ingestion including herbal remedies and alcohol intake, and blood tests should be taken to exclude superadded viral hepatitis (hepatitis A, C, D and E, CMV, EBV, HSV) and autoimmune hepatitis. A liver ultrasound should be performed to exclude biliary disease and to check that hepatic vessels are patent.

There is no history of drug or toxin ingestion, other viral serology and the autoimmune profile are negative, and a liver ultrasound is normal. Hepatitis B serology reveals that she is still HBeAg positive and her HBV DNA titre remains

Table 15.3 Serological markers for HBV infection.

	HBsAg	HBeAg	Anti-HBc IgM	Anti-HBc IgG	Anti-HBe	Anti-HBs	HBV DNA
Acute HBV							
Early phase	+	+	+	−	−	−	+
Recovery	−	−	−	+	+	+	−
Chronic HBV							
Immunotolerant phase	+	+	−	+	−	−	+
Non-replicative phase	+	−	−	+	+	−	−
Pre-core mutant	+	−	−	+	+	−	+
Vaccinated	−	−	−	−	−	+	−

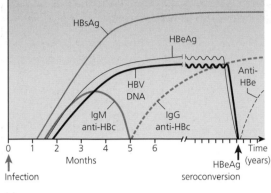

(a)

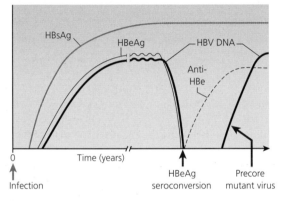

(b)

Figure 15.3 Serological changes in chronic HBV infection: (a) with HBeAg seroconversion, and (b) with HBeAg negative disease with development of a precore mutant virus.

high. Her hepatologist is concerned and organises for her to have a liver biopsy which shows active necroinflammation within the liver and early fibrosis.

What treatments are available to treat chronic hepatitis B infection?

• *Interferons*: These are naturally occurring cytokines that have antiviral, immunomodulatory and antiproliferative effects. They are given for a finite period, usually a year, with the aim of boosting the body's antiviral immune response, achieving HBeAg seroconversion and loss of HBV DNA from the serum. This occurs in about 40% of patients. A small proportion of patients (3-9%) completely clear the virus and lose HBsAg. Interferon has to be given by subcutaneous injection and its use is associated with significant side effects particularly flu-like symptoms and bone marrow toxicity.

• *Nucleoside/nucleotide analogues*: These orally active drugs work by inhibiting the viral DNA polymerase. They are incorporated into the viral nucleic acid causing chain termination. They are generally safe with a low incidence of side effects but viral reactivation usually occurs on stopping the drugs and their use can be associated with the development of antiviral resistance.

Amy undergoes a year of interferon treatment, which she tolerates well. At the end of treatment her liver function tests have normalised, HBV DNA is undetectable, HBeAg is negative and she has produced anti-HBe. She is monitored regularly in the clinic. At her follow-up appointment 2 years later she remains asymptomatic but blood tests are abnormal:

Bilirubin	*16 μmol/L*
ALT	*104 iU/L*
ALP	*74 iU/L*
HBeAg	*Negative*
Anti-HBe	*Positive*
HBV DNA	*Positive, 10^5 iU/mL*

What has happened now?

She has developed active HBV replication again despite being HBeAg negative and anti-HBe positive (Fig. 15.3b). This occurs due to a mutation in the pre-core region of the virus that permits viral replication even without HBeAg positivity. If untreated she will be at high risk of developing progressive liver disease and ultimately cirrhosis.

She is established on oral antiviral treatment with the nucleotide analogue tenofovir. Over the next year her ALT normalises, her HBV DNA becomes undetectable and she remains well.

CASE REVIEW

Tom Wong presented with acute hepatitis and serological evidence of recently acquired HBV infection. He was jaundiced and unwell but rapidly improved and cleared the HBV infection. Screening of his contacts revealed that his pregnant wife, Amy, was a chronic carrier of HBV. She was in the immunotolerant phase of the illness and was very well. She was, however, HBeAg positive with a high level of HBV DNA in the blood and therefore highly infectious and at particular risk of passing on the virus to her baby. The baby received a combination of passive and active immunisation which successfully prevented infection.

Amy subsequently developed a flare of hepatitis and required treatment with interferon. She seroconverted to anti-HBe with normalisation of liver function tests and loss of HBV DNA from the blood. Two years later, however, the HBV DNA became positive again despite the absence of HBeAg indicating that she had developed a pre-core mutant virus. She was treated with an orally active antiviral agent that controlled HBV replication.

KEY POINTS

- Hepatitis B infection is very common worldwide
- HBV is spread parenterally; vertical transmission is the commonest mode of transmission worldwide
- Acute infection is frequently asymptomatic but a few may develop a jaundiced illness. Liver failure does occur but is very rare
- The best test for acute HBV infection is to look for the presence of IgM anti-HBc
- HBV is a notifiable disease and all possible contacts should be screened, particularly sexual partners, first-degree relatives and household contacts
- Chronic HBV infection is usually asymptomatic

- In the immunotolerant phase patients have high levels of viral replication (HBeAg positive, high levels of HBV DNA) but poor immune responses to the virus. They are well with normal ALT but are highly infectious
- In the immune reactivation phase the immune response results in necroinflammation in the liver. This can lead to fibrosis and ultimately progression to cirrhosis
- HBeAg-negative patients can still develop viral replication if they develop a mutation in the precore coding region
- Antiviral treatment is available in the form of interferon injections or orally active antiviral drugs

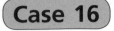
Case 16 Acute deterioration in a 21-year-old man with chronic hepatitis B virus infection

Benno Florio is a 21-year-old Italian university student who is known to be a chronic carrier of hepatitis B virus. He has never required treatment. He has a somewhat reckless lifestyle and occasionally uses intravenous drugs at parties with his university friends. He has become unwell in the past 2 weeks and is now jaundiced with tender hepatomegaly. His blood tests reveal:

Bilirubin	214 μmol/L
ALT	875 iU/L
ALP	142 iU/L
INR	1.1
HBsAg	Positive
Anti-HBc IgM	Negative
HBeAg	Positive
Anti-HBe	Negative
HBV DNA	Negative

What is the most likely diagnosis?

He has severe hepatitis and is a chronic carrier of hepatitis B virus (HBV). His HBV DNA levels are negative, however, making it unlikely that HBV infection is the cause of his deterioration. The most likely explanation is that he has acquired another hepatitis virus on top of his chronic hepatitis B infection. With his history of intravenous drug use hepatitis C or D superinfection is most likely.

Serology tests reveal that he is HCV antibody negative but HDV antibody positive with positive HDV RNA.

What is hepatitis D virus?

Hepatitis D virus (HDV or delta virus) is a subviral particle that is incapable of independent existence. It requires the presence of HBV to complete virion assembly as it utilises HBsAg to form its outer coat. As a result, HDV infection only occurs in combination with HBV infec-

tion. Active HBV replication is reduced by delta infection and patients are usually negative for HBV DNA. HDV infection is particularly seen in intravenous drug users but can affect all risk groups for HBV infection.

What types of infection can HDV cause?

• *Coinfection of HDV and HBV at the same time*: This usually produces a syndrome that is clinically indistinguishable from acute HBV infection. The diagnosis is confirmed by finding serum IgM anti-δ and IgM anti-HBc. The infection is usually transient and self-limiting although an increased incidence of acute liver failure has been reported.

• *Superinfection*: This occurs when a patient who is already suffering from chronic HBV infection acquires a superadded HDV infection. This typically results in an acute flare of previous chronic HBV and can produce an unusually severe hepatitis. Diagnosis is confirmed by finding IgM anti-δ at the same time as IgG anti-HBc. Following superinfection, progression to chronic HDV infection is almost invariable.

• *Chronic HDV infection*: This is a severe form of liver disease that rarely resolves spontaneously; 60–70% of patients will progress to cirrhosis. It is characterised by detection of HDV RNA in the serum.

How can chronic HDV infection be treated?

Interferon is the only treatment available for chronic HDV infection. The main goals are eradication of both HBV and HDV. Whilst it may control HDV replication, relapse is frequent when treatment is discontinued.

Benno is started on interferon treatment. He initially improves with a reduction in his ALT and bilirubin but a follow-up biopsy shows that he has developed cirrhosis. His condition gradually deteriorates over the next few years with progressive liver failure and development of ascites. He is referred to his local liver transplant unit and successfully

Hepatology: Clinical Cases Uncovered, 1st edition. © Kathryn Nash and Indra Neil Guha. Published 2011 by Blackwell Publishing Ltd.

undergoes liver transplantation. Following his transplant he is treated with hepatitis B immunoglobulin and antiviral agents which successfully prevent HBV infection of the new liver.

CASE REVIEW

Benno Florio is a chronic carrier of hepatitis B virus. He developed a superadded hepatitis D virus infection probably via shared needles used for administering intravenous drugs. He developed a severe acute hepatitis with jaundice. Although he improved initially with interferon therapy, he progressed to cirrhosis with decompensation requiring liver transplantation.

KEY POINTS

- Hepatitis D virus is a subviral particle incapable of independent existence
- HDV infection can only occur in patients who have HBV infection
- Co-infection occurs when both HBV and HDV are acquired at the same time. Infection is usually transient
- Superinfection occurs when a patient already harbouring HBV acquires HDV. It is associated with a severe hepatitis and high risk of progression to cirrhosis
- Interferon is the most appropriate treatment for symptomatic chronic HDV infection
- If a patient with chronic HBV deteriorates, superadded HDV infection should always be considered

Case 17 A 53-year-old man with a history of high alcohol intake

Ben Smith, a 53-year-old bank manager is taken to his GP by his wife. He lost his job 18 months ago and his wife has become increasingly concerned about his alcohol intake. He has always had a glass of whisky at night but his wife thinks he has been drinking more lately and has even found him having a drink in the morning to calm his nerves. He denies that there is a problem but his wife is worried that his high alcohol intake may be damaging his health.

On examination he has a plethoric complexion and bilateral Dupuytren's contracture. There are no other peripheral stigmata of chronic liver disease. His liver is palpable 3 cm below the costal margin but is non-tender and the rest of the abdominal examination is normal.

What questions would you ask him?

It is important to try to ascertain how much alcohol he is drinking. This is often a very sensitive subject and patients may not tell the whole story. You should ask open questions at first but follow up with more specific questions to determine the exact pattern of his drinking. Ask questions such as:

- What type of alcohol is drunk (beer, wine, spirits)?
- What percentage of alcohol does it contain?
- How many drinks a day or week? Patients often underestimate this so it is helpful to ask in several ways, for example enquiring about how long a bottle of whisky lasts, are the measures poured at home (drinks poured at home are often larger than those in a pub).
- How long have they been drinking at this level?
- What is the pattern of drinking (in the pub with friends, at home alone, etc.)?

It is also important to try to assess the degree of alcohol dependency and willingness to change. The simple 'CAGE' questionnaire is a useful screening tool to identify patients with alcohol dependency (Box 17.1).

What investigations would you do in general practice?
Laboratory tests

Laboratory abnormalities that may be associated with alcohol-related liver disease are shown in Table 17.1. Whilst the presence of these abnormalities may be helpful, they do not correlate with the severity of liver disease and none of them are specific for alcohol-related liver damage. Furthermore, laboratory tests are often normal even in advanced liver disease.

> **!RED FLAG**
>
> Normal liver function tests are not necessarily reassuring and do not exclude alcohol-related liver disease.

Radiology

Abdominal ultrasound is the most helpful first step in the evaluation of patients who have suspected liver disease. It is important to look for features of liver disease and also to exclude other causes of liver problems (e.g. biliary obstruction, hepatic lesions). As with laboratory abnormalities it is important to recognise that a normal liver ultrasound does not exclude the possibility of liver pathology.

> **Box 17.1 'CAGE' questionnaire for alcohol dependency**
>
> - Have you ever felt you should **cut** down on your drinking?
> - Have people **annoyed** you by criticising your drinking?
> - Have you ever felt **guilty** about your drinking?
> - Have you ever had a drink first thing in the morning to steady your nerves or get rid of a hangover (**eye-opener**)?
>
> Two 'yes' responses indicate that alcohol dependency is possible and further investigation is required.

Hepatology: Clinical Cases Uncovered, 1st edition. © Kathryn Nash and Indra Neil Guha. Published 2011 by Blackwell Publishing Ltd.

!RED FLAG

Significant liver disease, even cirrhosis can be present despite a normal liver ultrasound.

Features that may be seen in alcohol-related liver disease include:
- *Fat infiltration*: The liver may appear bright compared to the surrounding organs suggesting infiltration with fat.
- *Cirrhosis*: The presence of a small irregular liver is suggestive of cirrhosis. Features of portal hypertension may be present, including splenomegaly, ascites and abdominal varices.

At first Mr Smith is reluctant to answer the GP's questions regarding his alcohol intake but after careful questioning he admits to drinking about half a bottle of whisky a day. He admits that if he doesn't have a drink he becomes shaky and sweaty and to avoid these symptoms he has been having a glass of whisky first thing in the morning for the past few months. Investigations reveal the following:

Bilirubin	16 μmol/L
ALT	85 iU/L
ALP	92 iU/L
AST	186 iU/L
Albumin	35 g/L
γ-GT	257 U/L
MCV	108 fL

His GP organises for him to have a liver ultrasound which demonstrates an enlarged liver with a bright echotexture consistent with fat infiltration. He is referred to a hepatologist who arranges for him to have a liver biopsy. This demonstrates hepatic steatosis but no evidence of inflammation or scarring (Fig. 17.1).

What is hepatic steatosis?

Hepatic steatosis is the name given to the accumulation of fat droplets within hepatocytes. Alcohol is an important cause, but it can also be seen in other disorders including diabetes and obesity. Alcohol metabolism results in decreased fatty acid oxidation and increased triglyceride synthesis resulting in accumulation of fat within the liver, mainly in zone 3 hepatocytes.

Table 17.1 Laboratory abnormalities associated with alcohol-related liver disease.

Laboratory abnormality	Notes
Transaminases	AST is frequently mildly elevated (2–5 times normal) in alcohol-related liver disease
	ALT levels may be elevated but often to a lesser degree than AST. The presence of high transaminases (>300 iU/L) is not typical of alcohol-related liver disease and should prompt investigation for other causes of liver damage
Alkaline phosphatase	Levels are often normal or minimally elevated
Bilirubin	Elevated bilirubin in alcohol-related liver damage is a marker of severe disease, either alcoholic hepatitis or advanced cirrhosis
Macrocytosis	Seen in approximately 75% of heavy drinkers irrespective of the presence of liver disease. Folate deficiency may also be present, further increasing the mean corpuscular volume
Gamma glutamyl transferase (γ-GT)	Commonly elevated in heavy drinkers even in the absence of liver disease as the enzyme is induced by alcohol. Levels return to normal within a few weeks of alcohol abstinence. Also elevated by other enzyme inducers, e.g. phenytoin
Prothrombin time	Impaired coagulation is a marker of severe liver dysfunction
Albumin	Levels fall in severe liver disease
IgA	Serum IgA levels are often elevated in patients with liver disease caused by alcohol and do not always fall when alcohol intake ceases
Alcohol	Alcohol levels in the blood can be assessed and are sometimes used to assess compliance with abstinence

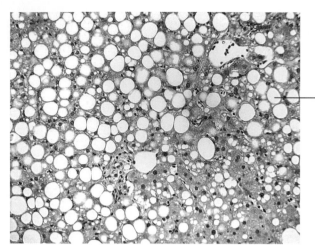

Fat accumulation within hepatocytes

Figure 17.1 Simple steatosis in this patient, evidenced by widespread globules of fat accumulation distending the affected hepatocytes. (Haematoxylin and eosin stain.)

What should the patient be told?
• His liver disease is fully reversible at this point. If he stops drinking the steatosis will resolve and he will have a normal prognosis from the point of view of his liver.
• He should be warned that if he continues to drink he could be at risk of developing progressive liver disease.
• He should be encouraged to stop drinking. This needs to be managed carefully in conjunction with an alcohol support network due to the risks of alcohol withdrawal if drinking is abruptly stopped.

What other effects does alcohol have on the body?
Excess consumption of alcohol can result in physical damage to a variety of other organs in the body (Table 17.2).

> Mr Smith is put in contact with the local alcohol support agency. He attends an initial consultation but doesn't return for any of the follow-up appointments. Six months later his wife takes him back to the GP with a 2-week history of increasing jaundice associated with dark urine. Examination reveals that he has lost a considerable amount of weight; he is jaundiced and has florid spider naevi over his upper limbs and neck. Abdominal examination reveals that his liver is enlarged 5 cm below the costal margin and there is a moderate amount of ascites. His GP refers him to hospital.
> Blood tests are taken and the results are as follows:

Bilirubin	389 μmol/L
ALT	57 iU/L
ALP	178 iU/L
Albumin	24 g/L
INR	2.2
CRP	68 mg/L

A liver biopsy is performed (Fig. 17.2).

What is the most likely diagnosis now?
The history suggests that he has developed an episode of acute alcoholic hepatitis, a condition characterised by intense inflammation within the liver (Box 17.2). The clinical features are of malaise, anorexia, nausea and vomiting which often leads the patient to stop alcohol intake a few weeks prior to admission to hospital. Patients are usually jaundiced and often have florid stigmata of chronic liver disease, particularly palmar erythema and spider naevi. There may be ascites and encephalopathy.

How was the liver biopsy obtained and why?
The liver biopsy would need to have been performed by the transjugular route. He has deranged coagulation and ascites, both of which are contraindications to percutaneous liver biopsy.

Table 17.2 Effects of alcohol on the body.

System	Effect
Central nervous system	Wernicke–Korsakoff syndrome
	Epilepsy
	Polyneuropathy
	Cerebral atrophy
	Cerebellar degeneration
	Depression
	Dementia
Muscles	Myopathy (acute or chronic)
Cardiovascular system	Cardiomyopathy
	Arrhythmias
	Hypertension
Metabolism	Gout
	Hyperlipidaemia (particularly triglycerides)
	Obesity
	Hypoglycaemia
Endocrine	Pseudo-Cushing appearance
	Gonadal dysfunction – impotence, gynaecomastia
	Parotid swelling
Respiratory	Increased chest infections including tuberculosis
Gastrointestinal	Inflammation, e.g. oesophagitis, gastritis, duodenitis
	Peptic ulcer disease
	Carcinoma (oral, oesophageal, pancreas)
	Liver disease
	Pancreatitis
Bone	Osteoporosis
	Bone marrow depression with cytopenias
Pregnancy	Fetal alcohol syndrome

Box 17.2 Histological features of alcoholic hepatitis

- Hepatic steatosis
- Ballooning of hepatocytes
- Hepatocyte necrosis
- Mallory's hyaline or Mallory bodies (inclusion bodies in the cytoplasm of hepatocytes). These are commonly associated with alcoholic steatohepatitis but are not specific for the disorder and may also be seen in other conditions such as non-alcoholic fatty liver disease, Wilson's disease and primary biliary cirrhosis
- Inflammatory cell infiltrate (mainly neutrophils)
- Pericellular fibrosis, which may already have progressed to cirrhosis

---

Box 17.3 Features of the refeeding syndrome

- Metabolic disturbances that occur when a patient who is malnourished is given nutrition
- Patients develop fluid and electrolyte disorders, in particular low phosphate, magnesium and potassium
- Glucose and thiamine levels fall
- In severe cases patients can develop confusion, fits, coma and death
- Treatment involves correcting electrolyte disturbances and replacing vitamins

---

How should he be treated?

Alcoholic hepatitis should be managed in the inpatient setting. Other forms of liver disease must be excluded by history, examination, blood tests and radiological imaging. The priorities of treatment are principally supportive:

- *Nutrition*: Oral intake is often poor as a consequence of anorexia, vomiting and encephalopathy. Patients fre-

quently require nutrition supplementation, usually by nasogastric tube feeding, and there is evidence to suggest that nutritional supplementation improves outcome. Vitamin replacement is required, particularly vitamin B_1 (thiamine), to prevent development of the devastating neurological damage of Wernicke–Korsakoff syndrome. Patients should be monitored carefully as they are at high risk of developing the refeeding syndrome (Box 17.3).

- *Sepsis*: Bacterial and fungal sepsis is common and a frequent cause of death. The presence of fever, a raised white cell count and inflammatory markers should prompt a search for infection and consideration of broad spectrum antimicrobial treatment.

- *Renal failure*: Patients are at high risk of developing renal failure. Urine output and creatinine levels must be monitored carefully and fluid balance disturbances corrected promptly with the aid of a central line if necessary. The development of hepatorenal syndrome (renal failure

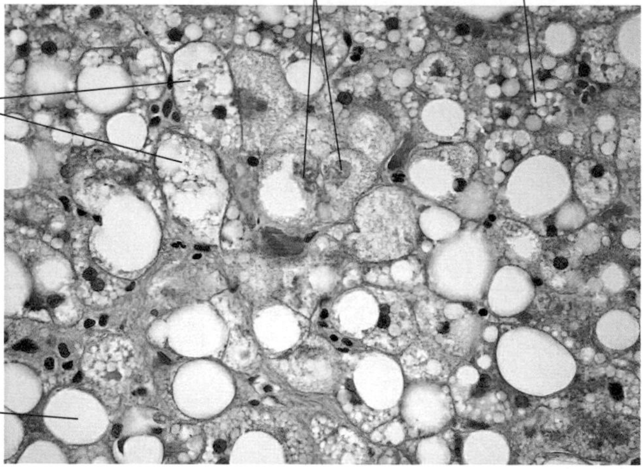

Figure 17.2 Liver biopsy in alcoholic hepatitis in this patient.

despite adequate central blood volume) carries a particularly poor prognosis.

Some patients may be candidates for specific therapy for alcoholic hepatitis. Corticosteroids are sometimes used but are associated with increased risk of infection and bleeding. Pentoxifylline, a potent inhibitor of proinflammatory cytokines especially tumour necrosis factor alpha (TNF-α), may be of benefit in selected patients. If the patient survives an episode of alcoholic hepatitis, support in maintaining alcohol abstinence is vital.

What is his prognosis?

In its severest form alcoholic hepatitis is associated with a mortality rate of over 50%. The condition often gets worse for a period of a few weeks after stopping alcohol. Death usually occurs due to sepsis or renal failure complicating liver failure. Most patients who survive an acute episode of alcoholic hepatitis and continue to drink alcohol will progress to cirrhosis.

He undergoes a paracentesis for his ascites and is started on nasogastric feeding. His condition deteriorates initially with an episode of chest sepsis complicated by renal failure and encephalopathy and his bilirubin rises to over 500 μmol/L. Following antibiotic treatment his condition improves and he is eventually fit for discharge from hospital 6 weeks later. He

continues to require drainage of ascites for several months but this eventually resolves. He attends regular follow-up with the medical team and the alcohol nurse specialist and manages to maintain abstinence from alcohol. Eighteen months later he remains alcohol free and has returned to work. A liver ultrasound demonstrates an irregular cirrhotic-looking liver but no evidence of ascites.

What is his prognosis now?

The most important factor governing his prognosis is whether he can maintain abstinence from alcohol. Despite the fact that he has cirrhosis his expected 5 year survival is up to 90% if he can remain free from alcohol, but falls to around 50% if he returns to drinking. Even with abstinence, however, a few patients develop progressive impairment of liver function or complications such as diuretic-resistant ascites or encephalopathy in which case they may be considered for liver transplantation providing they can demonstrate commitment to life-long abstinence from alcohol. Patients with alcoholic cirrhosis may develop hepatocellular carcinoma (HCC), despite abstinence, which results in death or need for liver transplantation. Therefore patients with cirrhosis regardless of abstinence should be entered into a surveillance programme to screen for HCC.

CASE REVIEW

Ben Smith presented with a history of high alcohol intake, features of alcohol dependency and abnormal liver biochemistry. At initial presentation he had alcohol-related steatosis, a reversible condition provided alcohol intake ceases. Unfortunately he continued to drink and re-presented 6 months later with the much more serious condition of alcoholic hepatitis. He was jaundiced and malnourished and suffered several characteristic complications of the disorder including sepsis, renal failure and development of ascites. With supportive care he survived and his condition improved; 18 months later he was still abstinent from alcohol. He had cirrhosis but his liver was functioning well, there were no features of portal hypertension and he was capable of holding down a full-time job.

KEY POINTS

- Alcohol is the most common cause of liver disease in the United Kingdom
- Hospital admissions and deaths related to alcohol use are increasing exponentially
- Excess alcohol intake can result in disorders of many different organ systems in the body
- Blood tests and other investigations can be completely normal despite the presence of advanced liver disease
- Hepatic steatosis caused by alcohol use is a totally reversible condition if alcohol intake ceases

- Alcoholic hepatitis is a serious condition with a high mortality rate
- Treatment of alcoholic hepatitis is principally supportive, involving improving nutrition and prevention and treatment of renal failure and sepsis
- Corticosteroids or pentoxifylline are used to treat alcoholic hepatitis in carefully selected patients
- Alcoholic cirrhosis may develop without prior symptoms of liver disease

PART 2: CASES

A 57-year-old man with diabetes and elevated alanine aminotransferase

Mr Michael Wong is a 57-year-old with diabetes who is found to have elevated cholesterol as part of his annual follow-up. He has been in the UK for the last 40 years having emigrated from Taiwan when he was 17. He was diagnosed with hypertension earlier this year and this is now controlled with an ACE inhibitor. The diabetes was diagnosed 3 years ago and has been well controlled by diet alone. The general practitioner discusses the benefits of starting a statin and measures some baseline liver function tests:

Bilirubin	*19 μmol/L*
ALT	*163 iU/L*
AL	*130 iU/L*
Albumin	*39 g/L*
HbA1C	*6%*
Fasting blood glucose	*5.2 mmol/L*
Fasting HDL	*0.8 mmol/L*
Total cholesterol : HDL ratio	*7*
Trigycelerides	*6.6 mmol/L*
Hb	*13.8 g/dL*
WCC	*5.2 × 10⁹/L*
Plt	*135 × 10⁹/L*

In view of the abnormal liver function tests the GP is reluctant to start the statin (a rare side effect of statins is liver failure) and asks for the patient to be seen in the liver clinic first.

How would you approach this case in the outpatient clinic?

• *History*: A detailed history should be obtained first. As well as a full general enquiry, information specifically relevant to this case includes:
  ○ Viral hepatitis is prevalent in South East Asia and a family history of hepatitis B should be specifically sought.
  ○ Alcohol history.

○ Drug history and in particular over the counter and herbal preparations.
  ○ He has some features of the metabolic syndrome (diabetes and hypertension) and associated conditions (e.g. cerebrovascular and cardiovascular disease) should be excluded.
• *Examination*:
  ○ Look for signs of chronic liver disease.
  ○ Take specific measurement of the body mass index (BMI) ((height in cm)/(weight in kg)^2) and waist : hip ratio as there are features of the metabolic syndrome.
• *Blood tests*: Chronic liver disease screen.
• *Imaging*: A liver ultrasound with Doppler examination of the portal vein.

Mr Wong has no history of liver disease and no family history or other risk factor for acquiring viral hepatitis. He is teetotal and the only medication he takes regularly is losartan 100 mg daily. He has not taken any other medication including herbal preparations. There is no history of ischaemic heart disease, cerebrovascular disease or peripheral vascular disease. His blood pressure is 140/90 mmHg, he has a BMI of 35 kg/m2 and his waist circumference is 110 cm with a waist : hip ratio of 1.5. The chronic liver disease screen is negative. A liver ultrasound shows an irregular margin to the liver which has a bright echotexture. His spleen is enlarged at 14 cm.

What is the most likely diagnosis?

The unifying diagnosis is likely to be non-alcoholic fatty liver disease (NAFLD) with underlying liver cirrhosis.

Mr Wong has a number of the features of metabolic syndrome:
• Insulin resistance.
• Hypertension.
• Hyperlipidaemia.
• Increased waist circumference.

In addition there are features that suggest he has significant liver disease:

Hepatology: Clinical Cases Uncovered, 1st edition. © Kathryn Nash and Indra Neil Guha. Published 2011 by Blackwell Publishing Ltd.

PART 2: CASES

• The platelet count is just below the lower limit of normal.

• There is an enlarged spleen and irregular liver margin on ultrasound.

A liver biopsy may be requested to confirm the diagnosis and the extent of fibrosis and to exclude a dual aetiology for his liver disease. The decision to proceed to liver biopsy, however, may vary from centre to centre. There is a growing utilisation of non-invasive markers of liver fibrosis (blood tests and liver stiffness estimation with elastography) and this is likely to change the management algorithm in the coming years.

What is non-alcoholic fatty liver disease?

• NAFLD is a spectrum of disease ranging from simple hepatic steatosis to necroinflammation (NASH or non-alcoholic steatohepatitis) to fibrosis and cirrhosis (see Box 18.1 for histological features).

• It is becoming the commonest cause of deranged liver function tests in the Western world. Population studies suggest the prevalence may be as high as 30% in the USA.

• There is a strong association between insulin resistance and obesity and NAFLD.

• NAFLD is a hepatic manifestation of the metabolic syndrome but may also aggravate and even initiate the metabolic syndrome.

Box 18.1 Summary of histological features that can be seen in NAFLD

• Steatosis
• Lobular inflammation
• Hepatocellular ballooning and Mallory bodies
• Perivenular/sinusoidal fibrosis
• Portal fibrosis (often seen in paediatric NAFLD)
• Bridging fibrosis

Box 18.2 Secondary causes of steatohepatitis

• Alcohol
• Drugs (e.g. amiodarone, methotrexate, tamoxifen)
• Jejunoileal bypass
• Parenteral nutrition
• Rapid, profound weight loss

• Only a minority of patients (approximately a third) with simple liver steatosis will progress to NASH and liver fibrosis. Presently it is difficult to know which patients will progress and it is an area of intense research.

• Secondary causes of NAFLD are shown in Box 18.2.

What are the management strategies for NAFLD?

• Lifestyle changes remain the mainstay of treatment for patients with NAFLD. Both attention to reducing calorie intake and increasing exercise is needed. If this is effective and sustained then improvement in transaminases are seen.

• Other features of the metabolic syndrome should be sought and managed appropriately, e.g. hypertension, hypercholesterolaemia and diabetes.

• In addition to the liver-related complications it is important to think holistically about patients with NAFLD as they are at risk from complications of coronary artery disease, cerebrovascular disease and both microvascular and macrovascular complications of insulin resistance.

• There is continuing research of specific treatments for NAFLD and emerging areas include insulin sensitising agents, antioxidants and bariatric surgery.

Mr Wong has a liver biopsy that confirms established liver cirrhosis with features consistent with NAFLD as the underlying aetiology. In view of the diagnosis of cirrhosis he undergoes a screening endoscopy that shows no varices. He is also placed on a surveillance programme for hepatocellular carcinoma with 6-monthly ultrasound and AFP measurement. The index ultrasound and AFP are normal. Mr Wong changes his lifestyle dramatically and loses approximately 15% of his weight by a combination of diet and exercise. He continues on the surveillance programme for the next year but following the sudden death of his wife he becomes very depressed and declines any further hospital follow-up. Three years after the diagnosis his family persuade him to return to the liver clinic. Mr Wong is generally well but has regained the weight he initially lost. His diabetes has become more difficult to control and he has been commenced on insulin. His liver function tests from clinic are shown below:

Bilirubin	*60 µmol/L*
ALT	*49 iU/L*
ALP	*209 iU/L*
Albumin	*28 g/L*
PT	*16 seconds*

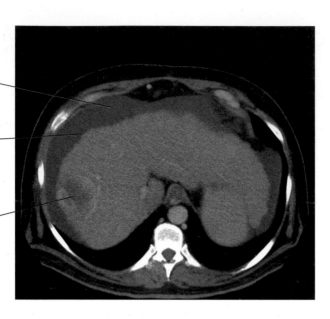

Ascites

Irregular edge to
liver suggestive
of cirrhosis

Focal mass

Figure 18.1 Hepatocellular carcinoma in
a liver with cirrhosis in this patient.

Should you be reassured by the fact that his ALT has fallen?

This illustrates the danger of looking at one liver enzyme in isolation. As cirrhosis advances it is not uncommon for the ALT to fall and a normal ALT is not reassuring. His liver synthetic function has in fact deteriorated as evidenced by his albumin falling, bilirubin increasing and PT increasing. The main possibilities for this are:

• Disease progression (from compensated cirrhosis to decompensated cirrhosis).

• Portal vein thrombosis.

• Hepatocellular carcinoma.

• Sepsis (e.g. spontaneous bacterial peritonitis if there is underlying ascites).

An urgent liver ultrasound is organised and this demonstrates ascites and a patent portal vein. There is also a 4.5 cm mass in the liver. A triple phase CT scan is organised showing rapid contrast uptake in the mass in the arterial phase and washout in the delayed portal phase (Fig. 18.1). The AFP is significantly elevated at 200 ng/mL.

What is the diagnosis?

Hepatocellular carcinoma (HCC).

What are the risk factors for developing this lesion?

• Liver cirrhosis is the most common reason for the development of HCC with over 80% occurring in this context. Malignancy probably results from continual cycles of inflammation and repair allowing cumulative mutations to develop in mature hepatocytes.

• The development of HCC is influenced by:

  ○ Geography (e.g. more common in eastern Asia and sub-Saharan Africa).

  ○ Disease aetiology (e.g. cirrhosis secondary to viral hepatitis, alcohol or haemochromatosis is associated with an increased incidence of HCC compared to cirrhosis secondary to autoimmune hepatitis).

  ○ Gender (males have a higher prevalence).

  ○ Age (may be a surrogate for duration of disease).

  ○ Activity of liver disease (e.g. HBV replication in chronic hepatitis B).

How do patients with HCC present?

Small hepatocellular carcinomas are frequently asymptomatic and only detected incidentally or by screening. Once the tumour becomes large it may cause symptoms (Box 18.3); by the time it produces symptoms it is rarely possible to attempt curative treatment.

> **Box 18.3 Clinical manifestations of HCC**
>
> - Decompensated liver disease:
>   - jaundice
>   - variceal bleeding
>   - ascites
>   - encephalopathy
> - Cancer related:
>   - weight loss
>   - decreased appetite
>   - malaise
> - Tumour rupture (haemoperitoneum)
> - Metastases
> - Paraneoplastic syndrome:
>   - hypoglycaemia
>   - diarrhoea
>   - polymyositis
>   - thromboplebitis
>   - hypercalcaemia

> **Box 18.4 Examples of interventional radiological procedures for HCC**
>
> **Transarterial chemoembolisation (TACE)**
> The hepatic artery is catheterised and then an intra-arterial injection of chemotherapy is delivered into the tumour vasculature (given in a carrier substance such as lipiodol). Following this the hepatic artery is embolised using an agent such as gelfoam (Fig. 18.2).
>
> Patients can experience post-embolisation syndrome (ileus, transient abdominal pain and fever). If these symptoms persist a hepatic abscess needs to be actively excluded.
>
> **Radiofrequency ablation (RFA)**
> Thermal injury is produced using an alternating electric current at a certain radiofrequency. The procedure can be performed by image guidance percutaneously or alternatively under direct vision at laparotomy.

How is HCC diagnosed?

The diagnosis is usually made by a combination of radiology (preferably at least two dynamic modalities) and AFP. Often HCC does not produce AFP and a normal AFP should not necessarily put you off the diagnosis if the radiology is characteristic. If there is diagnostic uncertainty a liver biopsy can be considered with the caveat of the risk of tumour seeding in the needle tract.

What are the treatment options for HCC?

Orthotopic liver transplantation

- This is the preferred option for HCC in cirrhosis because it also removes the background liver which is at risk of developing further tumours.
- Transplantation has a risk of mortality (less than 10% in most centres at 1 year).
- For transplantation to be considered the tumour should not have metastasised, should not have invaded the portal vein and should be within certain size criteria. These criteria are currently evolving but good outcomes are obtained if patients have a single tumour less than 5 cm in diameter or up to three tumours each less than 3 cm in diameter. If these criteria are adhered to, tumour recurrence following transplantation is low and 5-year survival rates of over 70% are obtained.

Resection of the liver lesion

- For patients with very stable liver disease and no portal hypertension or for those who are not liver transplantation candidates, surgical resection may be another potentially curative option.
- The selection of patients is important as the more advanced the liver cirrhosis, the greater the morbidity and mortality of the operation. Most centres would be reluctant to resect tumours in the presence of underlying portal hypertension and advanced liver dysfunction.
- The major disadvantage is that following the resection, the residual cirrhotic liver still has a propensity for malignant transformation.
- Five-year survivals may reach 70% in selected cases in high volume centres; the recurrence rate is also high.

Interventional radiological intervention

- A number of interventional radiology procedures are currently used for the treatment of HCC (Box 18.4).
- Whilst these treatments have been shown to increase survival, careful selection is again required. The presence

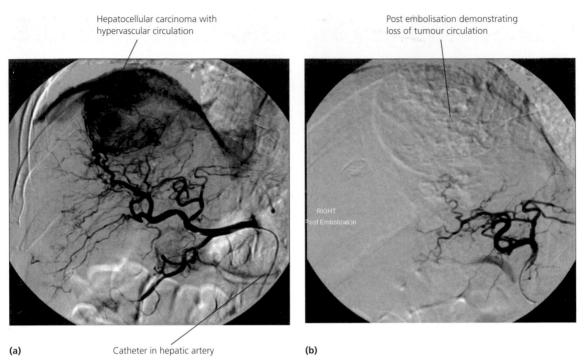

Hepatocellular carcinoma with hypervascular circulation

Post embolisation demonstrating loss of tumour circulation

RIGHT
Post Embolization

(a)   Catheter in hepatic artery   **(b)**

Figure 18.2 Transarterial chemoembolisation of hepatocellular carcinoma: (a) hepatic artery angiogram showing tumour circulation; (b) angiogram demonstrating successful embolisation.

of significant ascites and portal vein thrombosis will usually preclude radiological therapy.

• There is a growing role for using interventional radiology in patients who are on the waiting list for transplantation to keep control of tumour burden.

Pharmacological therapy

Novel agents such as tyrosine kinase inhibitors (sorafenib) have been shown to increase survival and their use is likely to expand.

Mr Wong was assessed for liver transplantation and accepted onto the waiting list; 4 months later he underwent transplantation. His ex-planted liver demonstrates a single HCC within a cirrhotic liver (Fig. 18.3). There was no evidence of vascular invasion suggesting a low risk of tumour recurrence. Three years later he is well without any evidence of tumour recurrence.

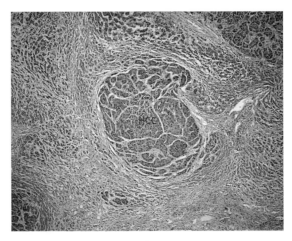

HCC

Figure 18.3 A nodule of well-differentiated hepatocellular carcinoma (HCC) arising within this patient's cirrhotic liver. (Haematoxylin and eosin stain.)

CASE REVIEW

A 57-year-old diabetic man was found to have deranged liver function tests during investigation of hypercholesterolaemia. He was found to have features of the metabolic syndrome and liver cirrhosis. A liver biopsy confirmed the diagnosis of cirrhosis secondary to non-alcoholic fatty liver disease (NAFLD). Surveillance for the complications of liver cirrhosis was commenced including endoscopy (varices) and ultrasound (hepatocellular carcinoma). Three years after diagnosis he presented with worsening synthetic liver function. Investigation, including dynamic CT and AFP, revealed hepatocellular carcinoma. He underwent liver transplantation and was well without evidence of tumour recurrence 3 years later.

KEY POINTS

- Non-alcoholic fatty liver disease is a rapidly growing cause of chronic liver disease in Western countries
- Features of the metabolic syndrome predispose to NAFLD
- There is a spectrum of pathology in NAFLD from simple steatosis to necroinflammation to fibrosis; liver biopsy remains the definitive diagnostic tool
- Liver cirrhosis increases the risk of developing hepatocellular carcinoma (HCC) of the liver

- Factors such as aetiology of disease, geography, age, gender and disease activity will all influence HCC
- Surveillance of patients with liver cirrhosis (using imaging and AFP) may pick up HCC at an early stage
- A number of treatments exist for HCC including surgery, interventional radiology, liver transplantation and pharmacological therapy.

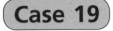

Case 19 A 42-year-old man with shortness of breath and abnormal liver function tests

Mark Simpson, a 42-year-old man, is being investigated by the respiratory team for shortness of breath. His breathlessness has been present for 5 years and is associated with a productive cough and wheeze. He is diagnosed with chronic obstructive pulmonary disease and treated with regular inhalers which stabilise his symptoms. During the course of his investigation he is found to have an elevated ALT of 120 iU/L. His respiratory physician organises for him to have a liver ultrasound which demonstrates a coarse echotexture to the liver with an irregular margin suggestive of cirrhosis. He is referred to the hepatology department for further investigation.

What would you do next?

As always, when presented with a new referral to clinic it is vital to begin by taking a comprehensive medical history. Enquire about specific symptoms related to the liver, past medical history, current and past medication and family history. A detailed social history should be elicited. A full physical examination should be performed; in addition to looking for signs of liver disease the cardiorespiratory and neurological systems should be assessed as they may reveal important co-morbidities or other clues as to the cause of the liver problem.

The ultrasound suggests that he has cirrhosis. Initial investigation should include a full chronic liver disease screen to look for the underlying cause.

Further enquiry reveals that he has been well throughout his adult life apart from the history of progressively increasing breathless. As a child he had prolonged neonatal jaundice which lasted for nearly 4 months but eventually settled spontaneously. He takes no medication apart from his inhalers. He used to smoke 15 cigarettes a day but stopped 3 years ago. He has never drunk alcohol heavily, consuming

Hepatology: Clinical Cases Uncovered, 1st edition. © Kathryn Nash and Indra Neil Guha. Published 2011 by Blackwell Publishing Ltd.

less than 10 units a week. There are no risk factors for him having acquired viral hepatitis. Further investigation reveals:

Hepatitis B and C	Negative
Ferritin	Normal
Immunoglobulins	Normal
Alpha-1 antitrypsin level	0.3 g/L
Liver autoantibody screen	Negative

What is the probable diagnosis?

He has chronic obstructive pulmonary disease, probable liver disease and a low α_1-antitrypsin level suggesting a diagnosis of α_1-antitrypsin deficiency. Other causes of respiratory symptoms and liver disease are given in Box 19.1.

What further investigations would you do?

- Alpha-1 antitrypsin phenotype.
- Liver biopsy.

His α_1-antitrypsin phenotype comes back showing him to be homozygous for the Z allele (PiZZ) confirming a diagnosis of α_1-antitrypsin deficiency. A liver biopsy is performed which demonstrates cirrhosis with globules in hepatocytes that stain with periodic-acid–Schiff (PAS) and are resistant to diastase, characteristic of α_1-antitrypsin deficiency (Fig. 19.1).

What is α_1-antitrypsin?

Alpha-1 antitrypsin is a serine protease inhibitor (serpin) involved in controlling inflammatory cascades. It is synthesised in the endoplasmic reticulum of the liver, secreted into the blood and transported to organs including the lungs. One of its functions is to protect the lungs by inactivating a variety of proteases including trypsin, chymotrypsin and elastase present in neutrophils.

The gene for α_1-antitrypsin is located on chromosome 14. Approximately 75 different alleles have been described, the most common are M, S and Z characterised by their electrophoretic mobilities as medium (M),

---

Box 19.1 Conditions that can produce respiratory symptoms and liver disease

- Alpha-1 antitrypsin deficiency
- Cystic fibrosis: respiratory symptoms predominate but patients can develop thickened biliary secretions leading to progressive portal fibrosis and eventually cirrhosis
- Hepatopulmonary syndrome: a complication of cirrhosis characterised by arteriovenous shunting in the lungs leading to hypoxia and cyanosis. Shunting predominates in the basal areas of the lungs and patients can exhibit profound desaturation on assuming an upright posture (orthodeoxia)
- Porto-pulmonary syndrome: a rare but serious complication of portal hypertension producing pulmonary artery hypertension, which can lead to right heart failure
- Hepatic hydrothorax: ascites may track into the pleural space producing a pleural effusion
- Cardiac disease: cardiac failure and pericardial constriction can cause hepatic congestion and be associated with respiratory symptoms related to the impaired ventricular function

---

Box 19.2 Genetic variants of α_1-antitrypsin

- PiMM — Normal genotype
- PiSS — Homozygous mild deficiency
  Produce about 40% of normal levels of α_1-antitrypsin. May be associated with liver disease if there are other co-factors, e.g. excess alcohol use or non-alcoholic fatty liver disease
- PiMZ/PiSZ — Heterozygote for deficiency
  Produce 40–60% of normal levels of α_1-antitrypsin. Liver disease does occur but is often associated with other factors known to cause liver disease suggesting that heterozygosity may predispose patients to cirrhosis in the setting of other causes of liver disease
- PiZZ — Homozygous severe deficiency
  Produce <15% of normal levels of α_1-antitrypsin. Patients are at risk of developing liver and lung disease
  PiZZ is present in approximately 1 in 2000 Caucasians, it is rare in black or Asian people

---

slow (S) and very slow (Z). The common genetic variants are shown in Box 19.2.

How do patients with α_1-antitrypsin deficiency present?

- *Neonatal jaundice*: Approximately 10% of ZZ homozygotes develop neonatal cholestasis with jaundice. Jaundice typically develops in the first 2 weeks of life and may be associated with hepatosplenomegaly. The prognosis is variable, and jaundice disappears in most infants after a few months but in some cases it may last for up to a year. Approximately a third of infants develop normal liver function, a third have inactive fibrosis and a third develop chronic liver failure and require liver transplantation.

- *Respiratory symptoms*: Patients with ZZ α_1-antitrypsin deficiency can develop panacinar emphysema and may present with symptoms such as breathlessness, cough and recurrent chest infections. Smokers tend to develop symptoms at a younger age (<40 years) and usually run a more severe course. SS homozygotes and MZ or SZ heterozygotes usually produce enough α_1-antitrypsin to protect the lungs from the effects of elastase in people who do not smoke.

- *Chronic liver disease*: 10–30% of PiZZ homozygotes will develop chronic liver dysfunction. Patients may present with complications of cirrhosis (e.g. ascites, variceal bleeding) or incidentally whilst being investigated for something else. Patients with cirrhosis are at risk of developing hepatocellular carcinoma.

What is the mechanism of the lung and liver disease?

A low level of α_1-antitrypsin allows unopposed action of proteolytic enzymes. In the lungs these are able to damage the alveoli resulting in emphysema.

The liver disease is not due to low circulating levels of α_1-antitrypsin since many phenotypes with a low or absent α_1-antitrypsin do not cause liver damage. Hepatic pathology is caused by accumulation of α_1-antitrypsin, probably as a result of misfolding of the mutant protein, which prevents its normal transport from the endoplasmic reticulum to the Golgi apparatus. The abnormal protein is visible histologically as intracellular globules when stained with diastase/PAS (see Fig. 19.1a). It is unclear exactly how the accumulation of these globules leads to liver damage; other genetic or environmental factors are probably relevant since less than 30% of individuals with the PiZZ genotype develop liver damage.

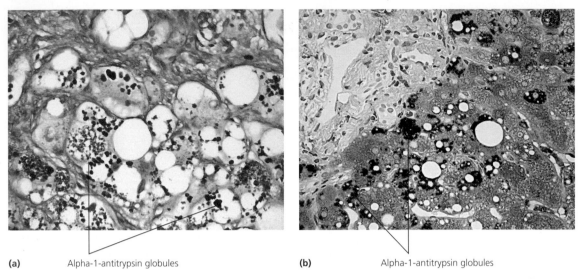

(a)   Alpha-1-antitrypsin globules   **(b)**   Alpha-1-antitrypsin globules

Figure 19.1 Alpha-1 antitrypsin deficiency in this patient showing prominent globules of abnormal α_1-antitrypsin protein accumulating within periportal hepatocytes: (a) diastase/PAS stains α_1-antitrypsin globules purple; (b) specific α_1-antitrypsin immunohistochemistry stains the abnormal protein globules brown.

What is the management of a patient with α_1-antitrypsin deficiency?

Management is largely supportive, including minimising the damage to the liver from other insults (e.g. alcohol, obesity). Complications of chronic liver disease should be managed in the normal way and patients with advanced disease should be considered for liver transplantation. All patients should be advised not to smoke to prevent or minimise lung disease. First-degree relatives should be offered screening and given lifestyle advice if found to be affected.

Mr Simpson is advised to keep his alcohol at a low level and to refrain from smoking. He runs an uncomplicated course and at follow up 5 years later has compensated cirrhosis and stable respiratory disease.

CASE REVIEW

This 42-year-old man was incidentally found to have an elevated ALT whilst being investigated for respiratory symptoms. α_1-antitrypsin deficiency was diagnosed by low serum levels of α_1-antitrypsin and cirrhosis was found on liver biopsy with characteristic changes of α_1-antitrypsin deficiency. He maintained a low alcohol intake and abstained from smoking and was well 5 years after diagnosis.

KEY POINTS

- α_1-antitrypsin deficiency is a cause of both emphysema and cirrhosis
- Homozygosity of the ZZ allele is associated with the greatest risk of disease, with 10–30% of affected individuals developing liver disease
- Milder phenotypes and heterozygotes may develop liver disease, particularly if other co-factors are present
- Liver disease may present as neonatal hepatitis or as cirrhosis in later life

- PiZZ homozygotes are at risk of developing panacinar emphysema, especially if they are smokers
- Treatment of liver disease involves lifestyle modification, management of complications of cirrhosis and consideration of liver transplantation if end-stage liver disease develops

Case 20   A 58-year-old man with diabetes and abnormal liver function tests

Mr Quentin Archibald is a 58-year-old man who attends the rheumatology clinic, complaining of pains in the small joints of his hands. He has experienced this for many years. In his past medical history he developed type 2 diabetes 5 years ago and has required insulin treatment for the past 18 months. He is not on any other medication. There is no family history of arthritis but Mr Archibald's father died of hepatocellular carcinoma at the age of 62. On general examination he is of slim build with a body mass index of 22 kg/m². He has a tanned appearance. There is 3 cm hepatomegaly but no splenomegaly. The joints of both hands are not hot or swollen but there is tenderness over the metacarpal joints.

Blood results reveal the following:

Bilirubin	13 μmol/L
ALT	124 iU/L
ALP	73 iU/L
Albumin	38 g/L

What is the most likely diagnosis?

Genetic haemochromatosis.

What investigations would be useful?
Blood tests

• Iron studies will confirm the presence of iron overload. Classically there is a raised ferritin and elevated transferrin saturation (often above 50%).

• An elevated ferritin may also be found in any acute inflammatory processes including acute and chronic liver diseases.

• A full chronic liver disease screen should be requested in case there is dual aetiology for his hepatomegaly.

• Inflammatory markers (ESR and CRP) and baseline investigations for an inflammatory arthritis (e.g. rheumatoid factor, anti-double-stranded DNA antibodies,

etc.) may be considered if the presentation is atypical but in the context of haemochromatosis alone will usually be negative.

• Genetic tests for haemochromatosis now exist and they should be requested in suspected cases. The two most common mutations in the *HFE* gene (C282Y and H63D) can be tested for.

X-rays of the hands

The arthritis associated with haemochromatosis is an osteoarthritis related to chondrocalcinosis. X-rays may therefore reveal degenerative changes in the hand.

Ultrasound of the liver and abdomen

• An enlarged liver can be caused by iron overload.

• Advanced liver disease, for instance cirrhosis may be suspected if there are radiological features of portal hypertension (e.g. reversal of portal blood flow and/or splenomegaly).

• In the context of haemochromatosis and cirrhosis, ultrasound is a first-line investigation for the surveillance of hepatocellular carcinoma.

What is haemochromatosis?
How is it acquired?

• Haemochromatosis is a disorder of iron homeostasis resulting in excess storage of iron in the liver and other organs including the pancreas, heart and pituitary gland.

• It is a genetic disorder with autosomal recessive inheritance.

• The *HFE* gene is the commonest gene involved and mutations in this account for over 90% of genetic haemochromatosis in European descendents. Homozygosity for the C282Y mutation is the most common and most clinically relevant abnormality.

• Having the abnormal genes for 'genetic haemochromatosis' does not automatically mean that individuals will develop clinical disease as there is incomplete penetrance. Clinical manifestations of the disorder or an

---

Hepatology: Clinical Cases Uncovered, 1st edition. © Kathryn Nash and Indra Neil Guha. Published 2011 by Blackwell Publishing Ltd.

elevated ferritin occur in less than 50% of cases with C282Y homozygosity.

How does haemochromatosis present clinically?

• Liver disease (abnormal liver function tests, complications of cirrhosis).
• Extrahepatic manifestations (Box 20.1).
• Clinically asymptomatic and detected by screening.

Box 20.1 Manifestations of haemochromatosis outside the liver

• General: fatigue, weakness, lethargy and apathy
• Endocrine: diabetes
• Hyperpigmentation: as a result of excess melanin deposition rather than iron
• Hypogonadism: may result in impotence or infertility
• Musculoskeletal: arthragia, arthritis (due to calcium pyrophosphate deposition in joints) and osteoporosis (hypogonadism)
• Cardiac: cardiomyopathy that can result in overt cardiac failure and arrhythmias

---

Staging of liver disease and hepatocellular carcinoma

• A liver biopsy is not routinely offered in haemochromatosis as the combination of iron studies and genetic testing may offer enough confirmatory evidence of the diagnosis.
• Situations where a liver biopsy may be considered is when there are very high ferritin levels (e.g. greater than 1000 ng/ml), clinical suspicion of severe fibrosis/cirrhosis exists or a dual aetiology (e.g. alcoholic or non-alcoholic fatty liver disease) is suspected. Furthermore, although genetic testing is helpful there may not be the facility to test for non-*HFE* genetic mutations in clinical practice.
• A liver biopsy can distinguish between true haemochromatosis (iron distributed in hepatic parenchyma (Fig. 20.1)) and secondary iron overload, e.g. due to repeated blood transfusion (iron in Kupffer cells).
• There is emerging interest in imaging techniques; for example MRI (with adapted software) can detect iron deposition in the liver.
• The importance of detecting cirrhosis in this group of individuals is for enrolment into surveillance programmes for varices and hepatocellular carcinoma.

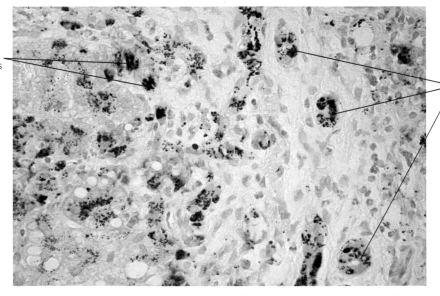

Iron in hepatocytes

Iron in bile ducts

Figure 20.1 Haemochromatosis showing marked iron accumulation within hepatocytes and the bile duct epithelium (Perl's stain).

How is haemochromatosis treated?

• The mainstay of therapy is regular venesection with the removal of a unit of blood, which contains approximately 250 mg of iron.

• By the time patients present with liver disease they may have accumulated 20–40 g of excess iron. It can therefore take several years of weekly venesection to remove the accumulated iron.

• The therapeutic target is to reduce serum ferritin levels to below 50 ng/mL. Once this target is reached venesection continues at a lower frequency to maintain the de-ironed state. Most patients in the maintenance phase require venesection 3–4 times a year.

• Chelating therapy (e.g. desferrioxamine) is not as effective as venesection but in patients unable to undergo venesection this is sometimes considered. The new oral chelating agents are expensive and are still being evaluated for this indication.

Mr Archibald's investigations return showing mildly elevated liver function tests, a ferritin of 600 ng/mL and a transferrin saturation of 80%. He is homozygote for the C282Y mutation.

He has a family with three children and asks if they need any investigation. What would be your advice?

Mr Archibald carries two abnormal copies of the *HFE* gene. Therefore all of his children will have at least one abnormal copy. If his wife is also a carrier (approximately 1 : 10 chance) then the children will have a 50 : 50 chance of being homozygotes. Therefore all the children should be screened for haemochromatosis with iron studies and genetic tests. There are psychological and potential financial implications of testing positive for haemochromatosis. Close liaison with genetic counsellors may be helpful in this situation. If the children are found to have genetic haemochromatosis they should be referred to a hepatologist for clinical assessment.

CASE REVIEW

A 58-year-old man presented with longstanding arthralgia, hepatomegaly and a tanned appearance. He has mildly elevated liver function tests, an elevated ferritin of 600 ng/mL and a transferrin saturation of 80%. Further tests reveal he has genetic haemochromatosis and carries two abnormal copies of the C282Y mutation. He is treated with venesection and his family members are screened for the disease.

KEY POINTS

• Haemochromatosis is a disorder of iron overload that results in excess iron accumulation in the liver which can lead to progressive hepatic fibrosis

• Haemochromatosis has a number of extrahepatic manifestations including diabetes, arthritis and cardiomyopathy

• Iron studies in combination with genetic testing may confirm the diagnosis

• Liver biopsy shows characteristic iron staining

• The treatment for haemochromatosis is venesection

• The presence of cirrhosis in the context of haemochromatosis is a predisposition for the development of hepatocellular carcinoma and these patients should be offered screening

• First-degree relatives of patients with genetic haemochromatosis should be offered screening for the condition

Case 21 — A 16-year-old boy with cognitive deterioration, ataxia and abnormal liver function tests

Brian Marshall, a 16-year-old boy, is brought to his general practitioner by his mother who is concerned about deterioration in his school performance. A year ago he was one of the best students in the school but since then he has had problems concentrating and his examination marks have deteriorated. His mother initially thought his change of behaviour was a feature of adolescence but she became more worried when his 10-year-old brother began to beat him at tennis and he had to leave his local football club as he was finding it increasingly difficult to run and control the ball.

On examination he is restless, he has an intention tremor and his movements appear generally uncoordinated. His speech is slurred. Cardiovascular and respiratory examinations are normal. Examination of the abdomen reveals a palpable liver and spleen. Initial blood test results are as follows:

Bilirubin	*15 μmol/L*
ALT	*102 iU/L*
ALP	*87 iU/L*
Albumin	*30 g/L*

What is the probable diagnosis?

The finding of abnormal liver function tests and hepatosplenomegaly in a young person with neurological symptoms is highly suggestive of Wilson's syndrome* (hepatolenticular degeneration).

What is Wilson's disease?

Wilson's disease is an autosomal recessive disorder of copper metabolism that results in abnormal copper deposition in various organs of the body including the liver and the basal ganglia of the brain. It occurs worldwide but is very rare, with a disease prevalence of approximately 1 in 30 000 and an incidence ranging from 5 to 30 per million population. The gene, *ATP7B*, on chromosome 13 encodes a copper carrier that transports copper between the hepatocytes and bile and enables synthesis of the copper-carrying glycoprotein caeruloplasmin.

What are the clinical features of Wilson's disease?

There are a variety of ways Wilson's disease can present (Table 21.1) and although the disease is very rare it should always be considered in a young person with cirrhosis or neurological symptoms as it is potentially treatable. Children usually present with hepatic problems which can range from fulminant hepatic failure to cirrhosis to being asymptomatic and detected during investigation of neurological symptoms. Young adults are more likely to present with neurological signs of basal ganglia involvement including motor disorders and behavioural changes.

Kayser–Fleischer rings[†] may be seen in the eyes of patients with Wilson's disease. They are caused by copper deposition in Descemet's membrane in the cornea and can be seen as greenish-brown discolouration around the periphery of the cornea. They are difficult to detect in dark-eyed individuals or patients with jaundice and are best identified by referring to an ophthalmologist to perform a slit-lamp examination. Despite their well-known association with Wilson's disease, Kayser–Fleischer rings are not specific for the disorder and can be seen in chronic cholestasis. They are not always present in the disorder and are frequently absent in those presenting with liver disease, particularly children.

---

*Samuel Wilson (1878–1937), British neurologist, who described four patients with tremor, dysarthria and movement disorders who were found to have cirrhosis at autopsy.

Hepatology: Clinical Cases Uncovered, 1st edition. © Kathryn Nash and Indra Neil Guha. Published 2011 by Blackwell Publishing Ltd.

[†]The German ophthalmologists Bernhard Kayser (1869–1954) and Bruno Fleischer (1874–1965) independently described the eye changes in two patients with neurological symptoms.

Table 21.1 Modes of presentation of Wilson's disease.

System	Clinical presentation
Hepatic	Acute liver failure with haemolysis
	Acute hepatitis
	Chronic hepatitis (vague symptoms followed by jaundice)
	Cirrhosis ± features of portal hypertension and decompensation
	Incidental finding of abnormal liver biochemistry
	Asymptomatic, noted during assessment of neurological case
Neurological	Deteriorating school performance
	Behavioural changes
	Psychiatric disorder (affective disorder, psychosis, dementia)
	Tremor
	Dysarthria
	Movement disorders
Haematological	Acute haemolytic anaemia
Renal	Renal tubular dysfunction
	Renal calculi
	Proteinuria
Skeletal	Vitamin D deficiency (rickets or osteomalacia)
	Osteoporosis
	Arthropathy

What investigations can be performed to attempt to diagnose Wilson's disease?

The most important step is to consider the diagnosis in the first place. No one test is diagnostic and there are numerous possible pitfalls in the interpretation of tests and the diagnosis of Wilson's disease. Investigations that may be performed are shown in Table 21.2. In patients presenting with neurological symptoms the presence of Kayser–Fleischer rings with a low caeruloplasmin are enough to make the diagnosis. For patients with hepatic disease the diagnosis is more difficult but is usually made if two of the following three abnormalities are found:

- Caeruloplasmin <200 mg/L (85% of cases).
- Positive penicillamine challenge test (>80% of cases). A 24-hour urine collection is performed after oral administration of the copper-chelating agent penicillamine. Urinary copper levels of >25 μmol/24 h are strongly suggestive of Wilson's disease (90% of cases).
- Hepatic copper >250 μg/g dry weight.

What is the treatment of Wilson's disease?

- *Reduce copper intake*: Avoid high copper foods, e.g. chocolate, shell fish and liver.

- *Drugs*: Copper chelators remove copper from the body, which is then excreted in the urine. Neurological symptoms can worsen when they are commenced.
  - *Penicillamine*: Copper-chelating agent with side effects that include skin rash, proteinuria, nephrotic syndrome and bone marrow depression.
  - *Trientine*: Copper chelator with side effects that are less common but can still occur.
  - *Zinc*: Reduces copper absorption from the gastrointestinal tract.
- *Liver transplantation*: All patients presenting with Wilson's disease and acute liver failure should be considered for liver transplantation if appropriate. Transplantation is also indicated in cases of decompensated cirrhosis.

Brian is diagnosed with Wilson's disease based on a low caeruloplasmin, positive penicillamine challenge and the presence of Kayser–Fleischer rings on slit-lamp examination. He is started on penicillamine which he tolerates without significant side effects. His liver function tests improve and 6 months later he has a normal ALT. His concentration improves a little but he continues to have a tremor and remains uncoordinated.

Table 21.2 Investigations for Wilson's disease.

Test	Notes
Caeruloplasmin	A low caeruloplasmin (<200 mg/L) is suggestive of Wilson's disease but pitfalls can occur: • It is an acute phase protein therefore levels may be normal or elevated in chronic hepatitis caused by Wilson's disease or if there are coexisting inflammatory disorders • It is synthesised in the liver therefore levels may fall in acute or chronic hepatic decompensation of any cause • Low levels can be found in heterozygotes • Rare, inherited deficiencies can occur
Serum copper	Serum copper levels are generally unhelpful. Levels may be low (if caeruloplasmin is low) or high (if copper is being released from the necrotic liver in fulminant liver failure)
Urinary copper	Baseline levels may be elevated due to increased clearance of copper, but the test has poor sensitivity and specificity
Penicillamine challenge	One of the most useful tests in the diagnosis of Wilson's disease Penicillamine, a copper chelator, binds to accumulated copper and is excreted in the urine A urine copper exceeding 25 μmol/24 h following penicillamine challenge is suggestive of the Wilson's disease
Liver histology	Many features are non-specific and non-diagnostic for the disorder: • Fatty change • Mallory's hyaline • Features of chronic active hepatitis, fibrosis or cirrhosis • Copper may be demonstrated by rhodanine staining in cases of established liver disease but this is also seen in chronic cholestasis
Liver copper estimation	An elevation in copper mass in dry liver specimens is seen in over 80% of patients with Wilson's disease The test is only available in a few laboratories and the liver sample must be sent fresh and not put in formalin
Kayser–Fleischer rings	Best detected using slit-lamp examination Absent in up to 50% of patients with hepatic presentation of Wilson's disease
Genetic diagnosis	Although the Wilson's disease gene has been identified, over 200 mutations are recognised and mutation analysis is therefore of limited value in primary diagnosis There is some role of genetic testing for family screening

What else must be done?

Wilson's disease is an autosomally recessive disorder, therefore Brian's brother is also at risk of having acquired the disorder and he should be offered screening. If he is found to have the disorder, treatment should be started before the onset of symptoms.

KEY POINTS

• Wilson's disease is very rare
• The disease results from accumulation of copper in various organs of the body
• The main modes of presentation are liver disease (typically in children) and neurological or psychiatric disorders (adolescents or young adults)
• Diagnosis of liver disease is difficult as individual tests have pitfalls and are not specific for the disorder
• Treatment involves reducing copper intake in the diet and drug therapy to eliminate copper from the body
• Patients with acute or chronic liver failure should be considered for liver transplantation
• Siblings should be offered screening for the disorder

CASE REVIEW

This 16-year-old boy presented with neurological symptoms and signs of chronic liver disease. The combination of these clinical features in a young person is highly suggestive of the diagnosis of Wilson's disease.

Hepatology: Clinical Cases Uncovered, 1st edition. © Kathryn Nash and Indra Neil Guha. Published 2011 by Blackwell Publishing Ltd.

Case 22 A 43-year-old man with a large gastrointestinal bleed

Mr Steve Ball, a 43-year-old man with a long history of alcohol abuse, was brought by ambulance to the emergency department having vomited several times. Soon after he arrives he vomits a large amount of bright red blood with clots. You are asked to assess him.

What are the immediate management steps?

When evaluating any unwell patient you should always begin with the ABC assessment:
• *Airway*: An assessment of the patient's ability to maintain a patent airway is mandatory and if necessary the airway should be protected either with a pharyngeal airway or tracheal intubation. Patients having a large haematemesis are at risk of aspiration. Furthermore, patients with liver disease may be encephalopathic or intoxicated with a reduced level of consciousness and unable to maintain a patent airway.
• *Breathing*: Oxygen saturations should be monitored and oxygen given by face mask.
• *Circulation*: The patient should be rapidly assessed for evidence of hypovolaemic shock (pulse, blood pressure, capillary refill). Adequate intravenous access should be established. At least two large bore cannulae are required to deliver intravenous fluids rapidly. Colloid and crystalloid should be administered in the first instance whilst further assessment and investigation is taking place.

What is the differential diagnosis in this patient?

The causes of haematemesis are shown in Fig. 22.1:
• *Variceal haemorrhage*: This man has a history of alcohol abuse and may have chronic liver disease, which can be complicated by portal hypertension and the development of oesophago-gastric varices.

• *Peptic ulcer disease*: Patients with high alcohol use have a high incidence of peptic ulcer disease and may bleed from gastric or duodenal ulcers.
• *Mucosal inflammation (oesophagitis, gastritis, duodenitis)*: Inflammation in the lining of the upper gastrointestinal (GI) tract is common in patients who consume large quantities of alcohol. This can bleed profusely, especially in patients with coagulation disorders.
• *Mallory–Weiss tear*: Repeated, forceful vomiting can lead to a tear in the mucous membrane at the oesophago-gastric junction, which can bleed. This is often seen in patients with alcoholism. Classically the patient vomits several times and towards the end the vomit contains blood.
• *Gastric carcinoma*: Cancers of the upper GI tract are seen more frequently in patients with alcoholism and these may bleed.
• *Other causes*: Other causes of upper GI haemorrhage include benign tumours, Dieulafoy lesions, aortoduodenal fistula, coagulation disorders (thrombocytopenia, warfarin) and congenital diseases (e.g. Osler–Weber–Rendu). Occasionally patients who are bleeding from their mouth or nose may swallow sufficient blood to cause vomiting and present with haematemesis.

> **KEY POINT**
>
> • A patient with alcohol abuse should not be assumed to have liver disease and be bleeding from varices. Other causes of gastrointestinal bleeding are also common in these patients

What are the important questions to ask?

• *Amount and type of bleeding*: It is important to try to estimate the volume of blood loss although the history often underestimates this as the GI tract can conceal a large amount of blood. Enquire about the amount of

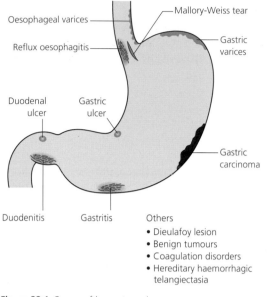

Figure 22.1 Causes of haematemesis.

bleeding and when it started. Haematemesis with fresh blood and clots suggests active bleeding in the proximal upper GI tract. Passage of melaena also suggests bleeding in the upper GI tract. Passage of fresh blood per rectum, haematochezia, in the absence of a lower GI source can suggest a torrential upper GI bleed.

• *Previous abdominal pain*: A history of abdominal pain may occur in patients who have peptic ulcer disease. However, patients can often present with bleeds from ulcers that have previously been asymptomatic.

• *Previous history*: Patients should be asked about previous GI bleeding and investigations and any past history of GI or liver disease or surgery.

• *Drug history*: It is particularly important to obtain a detailed drug history. Aspirin, non-steroidal anti-inflammatory drugs (NSAIDs) and steroids can cause mucosal inflammation and ulceration. Anticoagulation with warfarin rarely causes bleeding itself but can increase the severity of a bleed due to another cause. If patients are taking iron it may suggest that there has been chronic blood loss.

• *Alcohol consumption*: Alcohol use may cause liver disease with portal hypertension and varices. Patients who drink alcohol to excess are also at risk of GI inflammation, ulceration, carcinoma and other causes of GI bleeding.

What are the important things to look for on examination?
Signs of hypovolaemia

An assessment of blood volume status is vital to guide fluid resuscitation and to dictate the urgency of further investigation:

• *Tachycardia*: This is one of the first signs of hypovolaemia. Its absence, however, does not rule out a significant bleed since young, fit patients may have lost a considerable amount of blood before developing a tachycardia and patients on β-blockers may be incapable of mounting a tachycardia. Patients who are dependent on alcohol may have a tachycardia as part of the withdrawal from alcohol, which can be misleading.

• *Blood pressure*: The earliest blood pressure change of hypovolaemia is a postural drop. In a healthy person, however, over a litre of blood may be lost before a postural drop is evident. Supine hypotension may not occur until even larger volumes of blood have been lost. In contrast, the elderly may develop hypotension and a postural drop after much smaller volume blood losses. Blood pressure changes may be less reliable in patients with liver disease as they often have systemic hypotension as a result of the haemodynamic changes that accompany cirrhosis.

• *Peripheral perfusion*: An assessment of circulatory status can be made by examining end-organ perfusion. Cold extremities, pallor, delayed capillary refill time, oliguria and fainting or confusion suggesting cerebral underperfusion can all be signs of hypovolaemia.

• *Signs of liver disease*: Splenomegaly and ascites are signs of portal hypertension and their presence raise the possibility variceal bleeding. Variceal bleeding is the cause of bleeding in cirrhotic patients in 50–60% of cases but, as discussed above, patients should not be assumed to be bleeding from varices until this has been confirmed.

What blood tests would you organise in the accident and emergency department?

• *Full blood count*: In acute haemorrhage the haemoglobin is often normal in the first 24 hours, reflecting total blood loss. If blood loss has been chronic or occurred previously, the haemoglobin is usually low due to haemodilution by administered intravenous fluids and the body's physiological compensation by retaining extra fluid. Low platelets may suggest hypersplenism and portal hypertension.

• *Coagulation screen*: In liver disease there may be impaired synthesis of clotting factors resulting in prolongation of the prothrombin time or a high international normalised ratio (INR). This can increase the severity of bleeding and reduce the likelihood of it stopping spontaneously. Patients on warfarin may have a high INR and that requires urgent correction.

• *Urea and electrolytes*: An elevated urea may occur following an upper GI haemorrhage due to absorption of blood in the upper GI tract. Creatinine will usually be normal unless renal function is impaired.

• *Liver function tests*: Liver function tests are performed to evaluate the severity of the liver disease. Patients with an elevated bilirubin and low albumin may have advanced liver disease and be at high risk of mortality.

• *Blood cross-match*: Patients presenting with a large GI bleed should have blood cross-matched (4–8 units) and fresh frozen plasma and platelets available if appropriate.

On examination Mr Ball is pale and jaundiced; he has multiple bruises and spider naevi over his arms and chest. Whilst you are assessing him he has two more large vomits of blood. His pulse is 110 beats per minute and blood pressure 82/50 mmHg. His abdomen is distended with shifting dullness. Blood tests are as follows:

Bilirubin	217 µmol/L
ALT	46 iU/L
ALP	92 iU/L
Albumin	23 g/L
Hb	8 g/dL
WCC	5×10^9/L
Plt	34×10^9/L
INR	2.1
Urea	14 mmol/L
Creatinine	47 µmol/L

What emergency measures are required?

• Urgent resuscitation with blood to replace the blood loss.

• Coagulopathy needs correction with fresh frozen plasma and platelets.

• A urinary catheter should be placed and urine output monitored.

• Insertion of a central line should be considered to guide further fluid management according to the central venous pressure. This is particularly important in the elderly, who tolerate fluid overload or hypovolaemia poorly, and in patients with liver disease when overhydration may increase pressure in varices and exacerbate bleeding.

• The on-call endoscopist should be contacted and once the patient is cardiovascularly stable he will need emergency upper GI endoscopy. This is necessary to identify the cause of the bleeding and to apply endoscopic therapy.

Mr Ball is resuscitated and stabilised before being transferred to the endoscopy department. At fibreoptic endoscopy, a large amount of blood is seen in the stomach. There is no active bleeding but large oesophageal varices are present with red spots indicating recent haemorrhage. The varices are treated by band ligation (Fig. 22.2).

Why do varices develop at the oesophago-gastric junction?

Varices develop when there is portal hypertension. This occurs due to an increase in portal pressure due to either an increase in portal blood flow or vascular resistance or both:

$$\text{Portal pressure} = \text{Portal blood flow} \times \text{Vascular resistance}$$

Liver disease causes an increase in portal vascular resistance by obstruction of the venous channels in the liver resulting in increased pressure within the portal venous system. In addition, in advanced portal hypertension there is also an increased portal flow due to arteriolar vasodilatation of the splanchnic organs.

An increase in pressure within the portal venous system leads to the development of a collateral circulation diverting portal blood into the systemic veins via portosystemic anastomoses. At the gastro-oesophageal junction varices develop between the oesophageal branch of the left gastric vein (which drains into the portal vein) and the oesophageal veins draining into the azygos veins (systemic circulation). Other clinically important anastomoses occur at sites where the portal and systemic veins come together (Fig. 22.3):

• Rectal varices – anastomoses between the superior (portal) and inferior (systemic) rectal veins.

• Umbilicus – the recanalised umbilical vein in the round ligament (ligamentum teres) drains into the epigastric veins to form dilated varices over the abdominal wall (caput medusa).

• Stomal varices – collaterals can develop at the site of previous surgery such as around an ileostomy or colostomy.

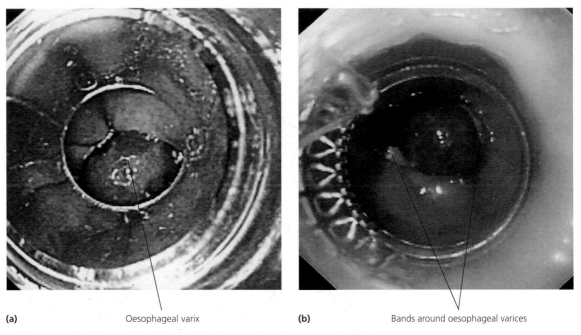

(a)   Oesophageal varix   (b)   Bands around oesophageal varices

Figure 22.2 Oesophageal varices viewed endoscopically before (a) and after (b) band ligation.

In health, the portal venous pressure is usually 4–8 mmHg. There is normally a gradient of approximately 3 mmHg across the liver from the portal (*c.* 7 mmHg) to the hepatic (*c.* 4 mmHg) venous systems; this is known as the hepatic venous pressure gradient. Portal hypertension occurs when this gradient exceeds 5 mmHg and varices may then form. Varices rarely bleed unless the pressure gradient exceeds 12 mmHg (Fig. 22.4).

How should bleeding oesophago-gastric varices be managed?
Endoscopic therapy

Endoscopic therapy is the most important step in the management of bleeding varices. Two approaches are available: sclerotherapy and band ligation.

• *Sclerotherapy*: This involves injection of a sclerosing material (e.g. ethanolamine) either directly into or alongside a varix and will control bleeding in 80–90% of cases. Complications include the development of oesophageal ulcers and strictures, oesophageal perforation, fever chest pain and mediastinitis.

• *Band ligation*: This has largely superseded sclerotherapy. The varix is sucked into a ligator, which is positioned on the end of the endoscope, and a rubber band is then placed around the varix (see Fig. 22.2). Banding and sclerotherapy are comparable in their ability to control bleeding but there are fewer complications with banding.

Pharmacological therapy

• Terlipressin is a synthetic analogue of vasopressin. It is a powerful vasoconstrictor, is long acting and can be given by bolus. It reduces blood flow to the splanchnic organs thereby reducing portal blood flow and portal pressure. It has fewer side effects than vasopressin but can still cause peripheral ischaemia.

• Octreotide is a synthetic peptide of somatostatin that causes splanchnic vasoconstriction and reduces portal pressure. It is virtually free of side effects but needs to be given by continuous infusion. If there is clinical suspicion that the patient might be having a variceal bleed then it may be justified to give pharmacological therapy prior to endoscopy since this will reduce portal pressure and permit earlier control of bleeding and may facilitate later endoscopic procedures.

PART 2: CASES

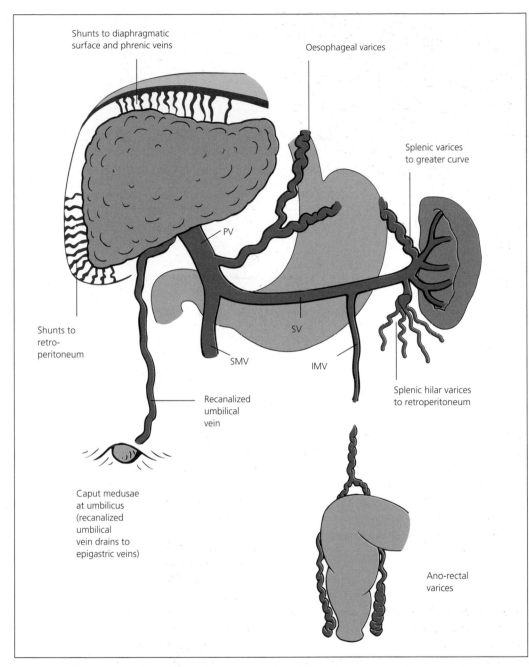

Figure 22.3 The sites of occurrence of portosystemic communications in patients with portal hypertension. IMV, inferior mesenteric vein; PV, portal vein; SMV, superior mesenteric vein; SV, splenic vein. (Reproduced with permission from Ellis H. & Watson C. (2008) *Surgery: Clinical Cases Uncovered*. Wiley-Blackwell, Oxford.)

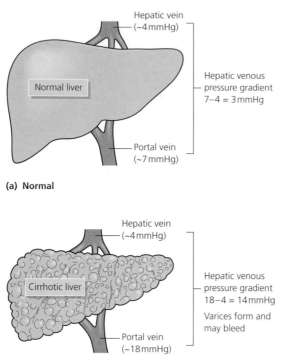

(a) Normal

(b) Cirrhosis

Figure 22.4 Development of portal hypertension.

What other management steps should be undertaken?

• *Antibiotics*: Approximately 20% of patients with variceal haemorrhage will suffer from an infection when they are hospitalised and invasive procedures will further increase the risk. Patients should receive prophylactic antibiotics such as third generation cephalosporin or ciprofloxacin as evidence has shown that they reduce rebleeding and mortality.

• *Lactulose*: Patients with liver disease who have a large GI bleed are at risk of developing encephalopathy. Laxatives (e.g. lactulose) should be prescribed to clean out the blood from the GI tract.

You are called by the nurses to talk to the patient's wife. She wishes to know about his prognosis. What should you tell her?

• His risk of dying during this admission to hospital is about 20%.

• Most bleeding can be stopped with endoscopy and drug management but patients remain at risk of complications such as sepsis, renal or liver failure.

• About 30% of patients will have an episode of rebleeding.

• Providing he survives this episode his long-term prognosis will be influenced most by whether he can abstain from alcohol.

Mr Ball initially makes good progress after his endoscopy. He passes melaena for 2 days but then his stools return to normal colour. The next day however he collapses on the ward after passing a large volume of fresh blood per rectum. He is resuscitated with IV fluids and blood and his condition is stabilised. He undergoes a further emergency endoscopy at which blood is spurting from oesophageal varices. Further band ligation is undertaken but the bleeding continues.

What measures are available if endoscopic and pharmacological therapies do not control the bleeding?
Oesophageal tamponade

Balloon tamponade aims to obtain temporary haemostasis by direct compression of the varices (Figs 22.5 and 22.6). It is rarely required nowadays due to advances in endoscopic and pharmacological therapy. Its main use is to gain temporary control of bleeding while awaiting more definitive treatment. A Sengstaken–Blakemore tube has two balloons, oesophageal and gastric. The lower, gastric, balloon is inflated in the stomach and the tube pulled back so that this balloon impacts at the oesophago-gastric junction. Compressing the varices here reduces flow into the oesophageal varices and in most cases arrests bleeding. Rarely, it is necessary to

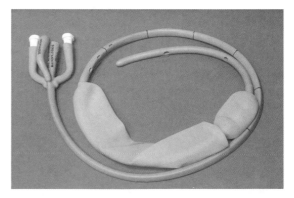

Figure 22.5 A Sengstaken–Blakemore double balloon catheter. (Reproduced with permission from Ellis H. & Watson C. (2008). *Surgery: Clinical Cases Uncovered*. Wiley-Blackwell, Oxford.)

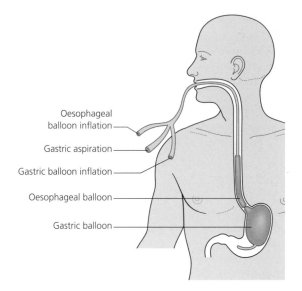

Oesophageal
balloon inflation

Gastric aspiration

Gastric balloon inflation

Oesophageal balloon

Gastric balloon

Figure 22.6 The double balloon catheter procedure.

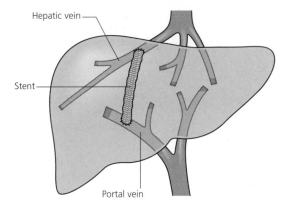

Hepatic vein

Stent

Portal vein

Figure 22.7 Transjugular intrahepatic portosystemic shunt (TIPS).

inflate the upper oesophageal balloon to directly tamponade the oesophageal varices. Whilst use of a Sengstaken–Blakemore tube may be life saving in cases of massive haemorrhage it is associated with serious complications, including aspiration pneumonia and oesophageal perforation.

Transjugular intrahepatic portosystemic shunt (TIPS)

Intrahepatic portosystemic shunting is now the mainstay for treatment of variceal bleeding where other methods have failed (Figs 22.7 and 22.8). Via a right internal jugular puncture, the hepatic veins are accessed under fluoroscopic guidance. A needle is then advanced into the hepatic parenchyma and contrast is injected to guide passage into the portal vein. The tract is then dilated and a stent placed. This acts as a 'bypass' for a proportion of the portal blood, resulting in a reduction in portal pressure and collapse of the varices. During the procedure the radiologist can directly access the portal vein and via this route can embolise the varices to prevent further bleeding (Fig. 22.9).

Emergency surgery

Due to the advent of TIPS, emergency surgery for variceal haemorrhage is rarely performed nowadays. Occasionally when a TIPS is not technically possible surgery is required. Most surgical procedures involve creating a shunt between the portal and systemic circulations to decompress the portal system, e.g. splenorenal shunt, mesocaval shunt or portocaval shunt. Alternatively, direct staple transection of the oesophagus may be performed to control bleeding. Surgery has a high mortality risk and following successful shunt surgery there is a high risk of encephalopathy.

Liver transplantation

Variceal bleeding is rarely a direct indication for liver transplantation but patients who have chronic liver disease should always be evaluated for transplantation.

Mr Ball is assessed by the critical care team, he is sedated and his trachea intubated to protect his airway from aspiration. A Sengstaken–Blakemore tube is inserted to temporarily control the bleeding. He is transferred to the radiology department where the interventional radiologist inserts a TIPS. This reduces the hepatic venous pressure gradient from 25 to 8 mmHg and successfully controls the bleeding. Following insertion of the TIPS he has an episode of encephalopathy that is managed with lactulose.

If bleeding is controlled after initial endoscopy, what should be done to prevent further variceal bleeding?

Following successful endoscopic control of an acute variceal haemorrhage, patients should enter into an endoscopic banding programme to eradicate varices. Repeat endoscopies with banding should be performed at 1–2-weekly intervals until varices are obliterated. This takes on average 2–4 settings. Following successful variceal eradication, patients should be periodically surveyed to ensure varices have not recurred.

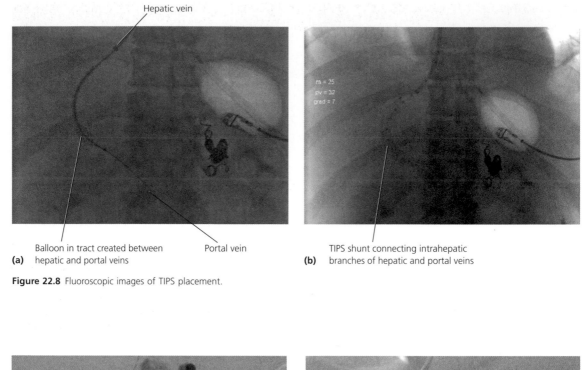

(a)   Balloon in tract created between   Portal vein
      hepatic and portal veins

(b)   TIPS shunt connecting intrahepatic
      branches of hepatic and portal veins

Figure 22.8 Fluoroscopic images of TIPS placement.

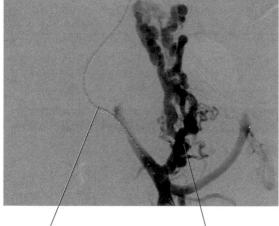

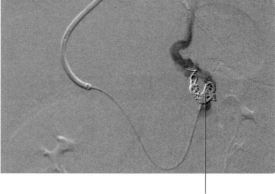

(a)   Catheter passed transhepatically   Contrast filling of massive
      into the portal vein   oesophago-gastric varices

(b)   Embolisation coils with dramatic
      reduction in contrast filling of varices

Figure 22.9 Direct embolisation of varices performed during insertion of a TIPS.

How could this emergency admission have been prevented?

Patients who are known to have cirrhosis should be screened for the presence of varices by endoscopy. If varices are identified then non-selective β-blockers (e.g. propranolol) should be prescribed to reduce portal pressure. If there are contraindications to β-blockers or these are not tolerated patients may have their varices eradicated by prophylactic variceal band ligation.

CASE REVIEW

This man had a long history of alcohol abuse and presented with vomiting and subsequent haematemesis. He was resuscitated with fluids and blood and his coagulopathy corrected with fresh frozen plasma and platelets. At endoscopy he was found to have bleeding oesophageal varices that were treated with variceal band ligation. This initially controlled the bleeding but he had a further torrential bleed requiring temporary insertion of a Sengstaken–Blakemore tube to arrest the bleeding. Subsequently, a TIPS was inserted that reduced the portal pressure and controlled the bleeding.

KEY POINTS

- Variceal bleeding has a high mortality
- Initial management is to secure and protect the airway and administer volume replacement to stabilise the patient
- Early endoscopy should be performed in patients with major bleeding to accurately diagnose the cause of the bleed and to permit therapy to control bleeding
- In suspected variceal haemorrhage, treatment with vasoactive drugs (e.g. terlipressin or octreotide) should be started as soon as possible, since a reduction in portal pressure is associated with a better control of bleeding and may facilitate endoscopic procedures
- There is a high risk of infection, and antibiotics such as quinolones or cephalosporins should be given
- Following successful control of bleeding, patients should enter a programme of regular endoscopy and banding ligation to eradicate varices
- If endoscopy is unsuccessful, patients may require emergency measures to control bleeding such as balloon tamponade prior to undergoing a TIPS procedure
- Patients with cirrhosis should undergo screening endoscopy to identify those with varices who can be offered primary prophylaxis with β-blockade or endoscopic therapy

Case 23 A 58-year-old woman with a distended abdomen

Mrs Anne Philly is a 58-year-old painter who presents with a 3-week history of abdominal swelling. On clinical examination she has stigmata of chronic liver disease (palmar erythema, spider naevi and caput medusae) and shifting dullness in her abdomen.

What are the possible causes?

This woman has signs of decompensated liver disease. Her abdominal swelling is likely to be caused by ascites rather than the other causes of a swollen abdomen (e.g. bowel obstruction, constipation, pregnancy). The causes of ascites can be divided into a transudate or exudate, defined by measuring the serum albumin–ascites albumin gradient (SAAG). A SAAG of greater than 11 g/L signifies a transudate and less than 11 g/L an exudate. The causes of ascites are given in Box 23.1.

What investigations would you do in a case of suspected ascites?

• *Ultrasound of the liver with Doppler examination of the hepatic vasculature*: This will confirm the presence of ascites (Fig. 23.1) but will also look for important conditions that can cause ascites, e.g. portal vein thrombosis and hepatocellular carcinoma.

• *Diagnostic ascitic tap*: This is mandatory in any patient with chronic liver disease presenting with new onset of ascites. Twenty to 30 mL of fluid should be aspirated using an aseptic technique and fluid sent for analysis (Box 23.2).

Why do patients with cirrhosis get ascites?

• The formation of ascites requires the presence of portal hypertension (Fig. 23.2).

• Accumulation of blood in the splanchnic arteriolar circulation is an initial event in the evolution of ascites.

It occurs due to an imbalance between local vasodilators and vasoconstrictors resulting in splanchnic arterial vasodilatation.

• This 'pooling' of blood in the splanchnic circulation results in a relative underfilling of the systemic circulation. The body compensates for this by increasing cardiac output and activating the rennin–angiotensin system to increase water and sodium absorption. Although total body water and sodium is high the amount retained in the central circulating volume is low and this accentuates a vicious circle.

• 'Back pressure' from portal venous hypertension and low oncotic pressure (reduced albumin synthesis), characteristic of cirrhosis, also contributes to ascites formation.

Mrs Philly has a diagnostic ascitic tap which shows an albumin of 16 g/L and a polymorphonuclear count of 50 cells/mm³. Her serum albumin is 29 g/L.

Is her fluid a transudate or exudate?

The serum–ascites albumin gradient is 13 g/L; therefore the fluid is a transudate.

How should her ascites be managed?
Bed rest

Bed rest can improve ascites as the upright position can result in activation of the rennin–angiotensin system, reduced glomerular filtration rate and sodium excretion.

Low sodium diet

The aim should be for a daily sodium content of 60–90 mEq. Practically, the advice to patients is not to add salt to their food and avoid processed foods. A balance exists between reducing sodium and making food tasteless so patients eat less and worsen their pre-existing malnutrition.

Hepatology: Clinical Cases Uncovered, 1st edition. © Kathryn Nash and Indra Neil Guha. Published 2011 by Blackwell Publishing Ltd.

Diuretics

• Spironolactone is an aldosterone antagonist and is the first-line diuretic used in cirrhotic ascites.

• The 'step care' management consists of increasing the dose of spironolactone and assessing response. There can be a delay of 2–3 days before the maximum response to spironolactone is seen. If ascites still persists, a loop diuretic such as furosemide may be added in addition.

• The aim is to reduce body weight by approximately 0.5 kg/day.

• Measurement of urinary sodium can help guide therapy.

• Side effects of spironolactone include hyponatraemia, hyperkalaemia and painful gynaecomastia.

• Renal function should be monitored closely as diuretics may precipitate renal dysfunction.

Box 23.1 Causes of ascites

Transudate
• Portal hypertension due to chronic liver disease
• Constrictive pericarditis
• Congestive heart failure

Exudative
• Malignancy including peritoneal disease and ovarian cancer (Meig's syndrome)
• Tuberculosis
• Nephrotic syndrome
• Pancreatic ascites
• Nephrogenic ascites
• Eosinophilic peritonitis
• Familial Mediterranean fever

Box 23.2 Diagnostic ascitic tap

• Position the patient in a lateral position and tap out the area of dullness
• Use a standard aseptic technique
• Using a green needle, aspirate fluid for:
  ○ albumin and protein
  ○ white cell count (with differential)
  ○ direct inoculation into blood culture bottles
  ○ LDH
  ○ amylase (if pancreatic source is suspected)
  ○ cytology

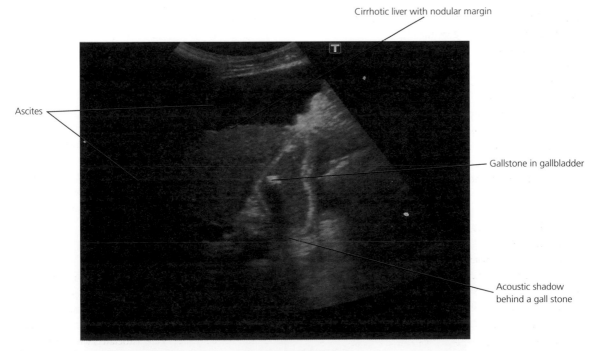

Figure 23.1 Ultrasound examination demonstrating ascites around a cirrhotic liver.

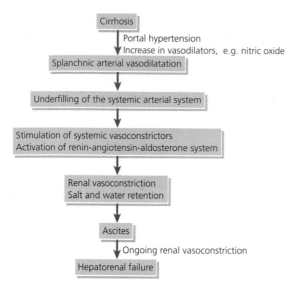

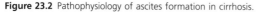

Figure 23.2 Pathophysiology of ascites formation in cirrhosis.

Paracentesis
• In patients intolerant of diuretics (usually because of hyponatraemia or renal dysfunction) or having persistent ascites despite adequate diuretics (refractory ascites), large volume paracentesis may be appropriate.
• Large volume paracentesis (LVP) involves removing ascitic fluid by drainage. The fluid should be removed over 6–8 hours and the drain removed to prevent the risk of infection.
• The removal of ascites can result in shifts of intravascular volume (post-paracentesis syndrome) and the risk of hepatorenal syndrome. Therefore LVP is performed with colloid infusion (usually salt-poor albumin) to maintain intravascular volume.
• The procedure can be performed as a day case.

TIPS and shunt surgery
• A transjugular intrahepatic portosystemic shunt (TIPS) is a recognised treatment of refractory ascites. It involves producing a shunt within the liver from the portal vein to the hepatic vein (see Case 21).
• In head to head studies of TIPS versus LVP there is equivalence of which modality is superior. However, with better selection of patients for TIPS and the use of covered stents it is likely the balance will swing towards TIPS in the future. The reduced need for paracentesis with a TIPS is countered by the development of hepatic encephalopathy in a small but significant minority.
• Shunt surgery is now rarely performed for ascites.

Orthotopic liver transplantation
• The occurrence of ascites signifies a major prognostic event in liver disease. The survival has been estimated to be 50% at 2 years and 20% at 5 years following the first episode of ascites.
• Consideration should be given for liver transplantation following the first episode of ascites.

Mrs Philly is commenced on diuretics and initially makes a good response to these. A transjugular liver biopsy confirms cirrhosis with a histological pattern consistent with non-alcoholic fatty liver disease. Six weeks later she is admitted to hospital as an emergency with abdominal discomfort and fever.

What is the likely explanation for her presentation now?
Her new symptoms raise the concern that she has developed infection in her ascites (spontaneous bacterial peritonitis). This can present in a number of ways including fever, abdominal pain, increase in ascites, confusion and worsening of liver function.

How would you investigate her?
A diagnostic tap of her ascites should be performed and fluid sent for white cell count and culture. Blood cultures should be obtained.

A diagnostic tap reveals a polymorphonuclear count of 400 cells/mm³. There are no positive cultures from her ascites.

How should she be managed?
• *Intravenous antibiotics*: A raised ascitic polymorphonuclear cell count (>250 cells/mm³) is indicative of spontaneous bacterial peritonitis (SBP). Ascitic fluid culture is frequently negative and the diagnosis of infection should be made on the basis of a raised fluid cell count. Positive cultures if available are helpful to guide antibiotic choice.
• *Intravenous albumin*: The development of SBP is frequently accompanied by deterioration in renal function, which can lead to the hepatorenal syndrome. Plasma volume expansion with human albumin solution (1.5 g/kg on the day of diagnosis and a further 1 g/kg on day 3) has been shown to reduce this risk and also reduce the mortality rate associated with an episode of SBP.

What management steps should be advised for her follow-up?

• *Antibiotic prophylaxis*: An antibiotic such as nor-floxacin 400 mg daily should be given as prophylaxis against further episodes of SBP.

• *Consideration for liver transplantation*: An episode of SBP has important prognostic implications, with survival at 1 year and 2 years as low as 30% and 20%, respectively. Therefore liver transplantation should be considered.

Mrs Philly is treated with intravenous cephalosporin and metronidazole and an infusion of human albumin solution. She makes a good recovery, following which she is assessed for liver transplantation and offered a place on the transplant waiting list. She is maintained on norfloxacin prophylaxis whilst waiting for a transplant.

CASE REVIEW

A 58-year-old woman presented with abdominal swelling due to ascites and decompensated liver disease. Diagnostic ascitic tap confirmed the presence of a transudate and excluded spontaneous peritoneal bacterial peritonitis. She initially improved on diuretics but suddenly deteriorated with an increase in ascites accompanied by fever. Spontaneous bacterial peritonitis was diagnosed based on an elevated ascitic white cell count and she was treated with intravenous antibiotics and albumin infusion. Once she had recovered she was referred for liver transplantation.

KEY POINTS

• The presence of ascites is a landmark event in cirrhosis signifying the transition from compensated cirrhosis to decompensated cirrhosis

• There are a number of differential diagnoses for ascites other than chronic liver disease.

• The management of ascites is a combination of diet, diuretics and paracentesis

• In more severe cases, radiological and surgical intervention may be required

• A diagnostic ascitic tap is mandatory to exclude spontaneous bacterial peritonitis in acute deterioration

• The development of spontaneous bacterial peritonitis has prognostic significance. Further recurrence is likely and therefore prophylactic antibiotics should be initiated

• Diuretic resistant ascites or the development of spontaneous bacterial peritonitis should prompt consideration for liver transplantation

A 67-year-old man with cirrhosis and confusion

A 67-year-old man with known alcoholic liver disease is admitted to hospital with confusion. He had been diagnosed with cirrhosis 3 years before when he presented to hospital with a variceal bleed and ascites. Following that he cut down his alcohol intake considerably but was still consuming two glasses of wine on most nights. He had had no further problem with variceal haemorrhage and his ascites was managed with a combination of spironolactone and furosemide. A week prior to his admission he had fallen at home, fracturing his right humerus and two ribs. He has been taking regular analgesia following the fall.

On examination he is disorientated and confused. He has palmar erythema and a few spider naevi. There is extensive bruising over his arm, neck and chest wall. His liver is not palpable but his spleen can be felt 3 cm below the costal margin and there is a moderate amount of ascites. Rectal examination reveals hard dark stools.

Investigations are as follows:

Bilirubin	35 μmol/L
ALT	45 iU/L
ALP	87 iU/L
Hb	8.5 g/dL
WCC	12.1 × 10⁹/L
Plt	94 × 10⁹/L
INR	1.7
Urea	12.1 mmol/L
Sodium	128 mmol/L
Potassium	3.1 mmol/L
Creatinine	105 μmol/L
CRP	85 mg/L

What is the most likely diagnosis?

Confusion in a patient with cirrhosis is most likely to be caused by hepatic encephalopathy.

Hepatology: Clinical Cases Uncovered, 1st edition. © Kathryn Nash and Indra Neil Guha. Published 2011 by Blackwell Publishing Ltd.

What other causes should be considered?

Encephalopathy is the most likely diagnosis but patients should be carefully evaluated for other causes of confusion, for example:

• Brain haemorrhage (in a patient with a history of excess alcohol intake and recent fall the possibility of an intracranial bleed, particularly a subdural haematoma, should be considered).

• Hypoxic/ischaemic brain injury.

• Infection (especially meningitis or encephalitis).

• Neoplasm of the brain.

• Drug overdose, alcohol intoxification and alcohol withdrawal.

• Metabolic disturbance (e.g. hypoglycaemia, electrolyte disorder).

• Endocrine disorder (e.g. adrenal, thyroid disorder).

What is hepatic encephalopathy?

Hepatic encephalopathy is the term given for the neuropsychiatric disturbance observed in patients with liver dysfunction. It occurs in both acute liver failure and also in patients with cirrhosis. The condition is usually reversible although chronic encephalopathy may be associated with irreversible brain damage. Several factors are thought to play a part in the development of hepatic encephalopathy (Box 24.1).

What are the clinical features?

Hepatic encephalopathy can take many forms and any change in mental status in a patient with known or suspected liver dysfunction should be considered to be due to hepatic encephalopathy until proven otherwise. Common disturbances seen include:

• Disturbed consciousness (excessive sleepiness, reversal of the normal day/night sleep pattern, reduced responsiveness progressing to coma).

• Confusion and disorientation (varies from minor impairment to gross confusion).

> **Box 24.1 Pathophysiology of hepatic encephalopathy**
>
> - Impaired liver function results in a reduction in first-pass metabolism of 'toxins' that reach the liver in portal venous blood
> - Portal blood rich in nitrogenous substances bypasses the cirrhotic liver via portosystemic collaterals and reaches the brain
> - An increase in 'toxin' levels in the systemic circulation (e.g. due to infection) increase the likelihood of hepatic encephalopathy

> **Box 24.2 Precipitants of hepatic encephalopathy in a patient with cirrhosis**
>
> - Constipation
> - Gastrointestinal haemorrhage
> - Infection
> - Drugs, e.g. narcotics or benzodiazepines
> - Electrolyte disturbance (hypokalaemia, hyponatraemia)
> - Dehydration (including that caused by diuretic therapy and abdominal paracentesis)
> - Uraemia
> - Portosystemic shunt procedures (surgical or radiological shunts including transjugular intrahepatic portosystemic shunt)
> - Portal vein thrombosis
> - Excessive protein intake
> - Superimposed hepatic injury
> - Any surgical procedure

- Disturbance of personality and mood.
- Flapping tremor (asterixis) may be present.
- Hepatic fetor.

These features may fluctuate and the patient can be completely well in between episodes.

What precipitating factors could be relevant in the case described?

- *Constipation*: Rectal examination in this patient revealed hard stools. Prolonged colonic transit time increases the toxin load in the portal venous system and can precipitate or exacerbate encephalopathy.
- *Gastrointestinal haemorrhage*: This patient has a history of previous variceal bleeding. At presentation he is anaemic with raised urea and dark stools on rectal examination, suggesting possible gastrointestinal haemorrhage. Blood produces a large protein load in the gastrointestinal tract and absorption of this into the portal venous system can induce encephalopathy.
- *Analgesic medication*: Opiate-containing medications may precipitate encephalopathy either by direct effects on the brain or as a consequence of their constipating effect.
- *Dehydration and electrolyte disturbance*: Cirrhotic patients are frequently intravascularly depleted; in addition, this patient is on diuretics putting him at further risk of dehydration. His sodium and potassium are low, both of which can contribute to encephalopathy.
- *Infection*: Infection is a common precipitant of encephalopathy and should always be considered and actively sought. This man's CRP is raised which could indicate an underlying infection.

Other precipitating factors for hepatic encephalopathy are given in Box 24.2.

How is encephalopathy managed?
Acute encephalopathy

- If the patient is in a coma, supportive measures should be instigated (e.g. airway protection, fluid balance, nutrition support).
- Identify and remove any possible precipitant (correct electrolyte disturbances, stop drugs especially opiates, benzodiazepines and diuretics).
- Actively seek and treat any infection.
- Empty the bowel of nitrogenous substances using laxatives (e.g. lactulose) and enemas. If there is gastrointestinal haemorrhage this must be treated promptly.

Restricting protein in the diet is no longer recommended as patients with liver disease severe enough to cause encephalopathy are frequently malnourished and in a state of protein catabolism. These patients actually benefit from high protein feeding.

Chronic encephalopathy

- Avoid precipitating factors (constipation, narcotic drugs, over-diuresis).
- Give lactulose 10–30 mL up to three times a day.
- Chronic encephalopathy may be an indication for liver transplantation.

A septic screen is performed and does not demonstrate any evidence of infection. At gastroscopy he is found to have altered blood in the stomach, severe oesophagitis and an erosive gastritis. He is treated with a proton pump inhibitor, his diuretics are stopped and he is given intravenous fluids and electrolyte replacement. Lactulose and phosphate enemas are given to good effect and his condition begins to improve. Thirty-six hours after his admission he becomes more confused and restless. On examination he is sweaty, tremulous and has a tachycardia of 120 beats per minute.

What do you think has happened?

His clinical condition now most likely reflects the alcohol withdrawal syndrome (Box 24.3). Alternative explanations should be considered including sepsis, gastrointestinal haemorrhage, head injury or metabolic disturbance such as hypoglycaemia.

How would you manage him now?

Box 24.3 Features of the alcohol withdrawal syndrome

This is a clinical syndrome that usually commences 1–4 days after cessation of chronic alcohol intake. Features include:

- Neurological hyperexcitability:
  - agitation
  - anxiety
  - tremor
  - seizures
  - confusion
  - hallucinations (usually visual)
- Autonomic instability:
  - sweating
  - diarrhoea
  - tachycardia

Managing the alcohol withdrawal syndrome is challenging in any patient but particularly so in one who is at risk of hepatic encephalopathy. The first priority is the safety of the patient and those around them. Patients can sometimes become aggressive and dangerous or may develop uncontrollable seizures; in these situations it may be necessary to sedate and ventilate the patient.

In milder cases, benzodiazepines such as chlordiazepoxide should be given. Small doses of an antipsychotic agent such as haloperidol may be required if there is marked confusion with hallucinations. In many cases, a reducing regimen of chlordiazepoxide is prescribed that tapers the dose over a 5–7-day course. Great care must be given in prescribing such a regimen in a liver patient as they are more susceptible to the sedative effects of these drugs. The prescription should be reviewed daily and adjusted according to the patient's clinical condition.

Patients should also be given intravenous B vitamins to protect against developing Wernicke-Korsakoff syndrome.

KEY POINT

- Patients with liver disease are very sensitive to sedative drugs. Prescribe as small an amount as possible, review the patient frequently, and adjust the dose according to the clinical effect

---

He is started on a reducing course of chlordiazepoxide which improves his confusion and irritability. This is discontinued after 5 days; he is much improved without any evidence of confusion and is discharged home.

CASE REVIEW

This patient with known cirrhosis presented to hospital with a history of confusion. The most likely cause was hepatic encephalopathy. There were several possible precipitants including dehydration, uraemia, electrolyte disturbance and gastrointestinal haemorrhage. His fluid balance and electrolyte disturbance were corrected and he was treated with lactulose and phosphate enemas with initial improvement of his symptoms. He subsequently deteriorated due to development of the alcohol withdrawal syndrome. He was carefully treated with a tapering course of chlordiazepoxide with resolution of his confusion.

KEY POINTS

- Confusion in a patient with cirrhosis is most likely to be caused by encephalopathy
- Other causes of confusion and coma must always be considered and appropriate investigations performed
- Encephalopathy is usually a fully reversible condition
- There are many possible precipitating factors that should be considered and corrected if possible

- Treatment involves removing any precipitant and encouraging bowel emptying with lactulose and phosphate enemas
- Alcohol withdrawal syndrome is a dangerous condition; patients should be managed on an individual basis with cautious use of sedative medication and involvement of the critical care team if the presentation is severe

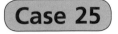

Case 25 A 47-year-old woman suddenly presents with variceal haemorrhage

Mrs Jackie Winter is a 47-year-old woman who presents to the emergency department with an acute gastrointestinal haemorrhage. She is resuscitated and an emergency endoscopy is requested. This reveals small oesophageal varices but large gastric varices in the fundus of the stomach (Fig. 25.1). She has no known history of liver disease. She drinks three glasses of wine a week and has never drunk more excessively. There is no past medical history of note and she is not on any medications. The following investigations return within 48 hours:

Bilirubin	*17 μmol/L*
ALT	*34 iU/L*
ALP	*78 iU/L*
Albumin	*40 g/L*
PT	*12 seconds*
Hb	*12 g/dL (post transfusion)*
Plt	*56 × 10⁹/L*
WBC	*3.1 × 10⁹/L*

Liver disease screen (HBV/HCV serology, autoimmune profile, immunoglobulins, α₁-antitrypsin, caeruloplasmin, and ferritin) are all within normal range or negative

What are the possible causes for her bleeding varices?

Varices signify the presence of portal hypertension. The causes can be divided into the anatomical site of obstruction/increased resistance in the hepatic vasculature. These are:

1 *Pre-sinusoidal*: Examples include:
   • Portal vein thrombosis.
   • Splenic vein thrombosis (gastric varices).
2 *Intrahepatic*: Examples include:
   • Liver cirrhosis.

• Schistosomiasis.
   • Nodular regenerative hyperplasia.
3 *Posthepatic*: Examples include:
   • Budd–Chiari syndrome.
   • Veno-occlusive disease.
   • Constrictive pericarditis.

How are bleeding gastric varices managed?

Bleeding from gastric varices is less common than oesophageal variceal bleeding but is more challenging to treat and is associated with a high mortality rate. The varices are generally large with a high volume of blood flowing through them. Band ligation or sclerotherapy with ethanolamine are not generally recommended as they are associated with a high incidence of rebleeding. Recently some centres have demonstrated success in controlling bleeding with an injection of cyanoacrylate ('superglue') directly into the varices. If bleeding cannot be controlled endoscopically, then the patient may require balloon tamponade for initial stabilisation (see Case 21) and then consideration for TIPS or rarely shunt surgery.

Mrs Winter undergoes a liver ultrasound with Doppler examination which reveals a portal vein thrombosis. The liver echotexture looks normal and the spleen is enlarged. A CT scan of the liver confirms portal vein thrombosis. There is evidence of collateralisation at the porta hepatitis (cavernous transformation) suggesting that the portal vein thrombosis is not a recent occurrence (Fig. 25.2). The liver looks normal but there is splenomegaly.

What are the two major differential diagnoses now?

• Cirrhosis with portal vein thrombosis.
• *De novo* portal vein thrombosis.

Miss Winter has normal liver function tests and the chronic liver disease screen is normal. This, however,

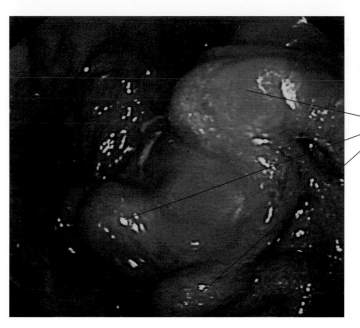

Enormous varices in the gastric fundus

Figure 25.1 Gastric varices seen at gastroscopy in this patient.

does not preclude the diagnosis of cirrhosis; as mentioned in other sections liver function tests can be entirely normal in cirrhosis. Against the diagnosis of cirrhosis is the fact that the portal hypertension is out of keeping to her synthetic function (normal albumin, clotting and bilirubin). To be certain that she does not have cirrhosis a liver biopsy should be considered.

> *A liver biopsy is performed and confirms normal hepatic architecture without evidence of cirrhosis.*

What are the possible explanations for her portal vein thrombosis?

The main causes of portal vein thrombosis are as follows:
- Liver cirrhosis.
- Intra-abdominal sepsis (e.g. diverticular disease or appendicitis).
- Abdominal trauma or surgery.
- Pancreatitis (may start as splenic vein thrombosis).
- Neonatal umbilical vein occlusion, e.g. by catheterisation or sepsis.
- Myeloproliferative disorders.
- Hypercoagulable disorders.
- Malignancy (HCC and pancreatic carcinoma).

- Congenital causes.
- Idiopathic causes.

What are the features of portal vein thrombosis?

- It can present acutely with right upper quadrant pain and fever but often the precipitant (e.g. appendicitis) will dictate the presenting symptoms.
- If there is mesenteric ischaemia due to complete occlusion this may result in an ischaemic bowel (abdominal pain, bleeding, lactic acidosis).
- Progression from the acute to the chronic phase leads to the formation of collateral vessels and classic cavernous transformation (recruitment of minor vessels that run adjacent to the portal vein and serve as a conduit of blood in obstruction).
- In the absence of underlying liver cirrhosis, portal vein thrombosis may not present with many symptoms until many years later; there is a buffering response with increased blood flow in the hepatic artery. The commonest presentation is with varices.
- In cirrhosis, a superimposed portal vein thrombosis can lead to decompensation with encephalopathy, bleeding, jaundice or ascites.

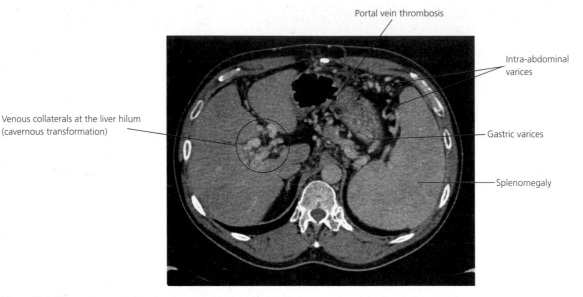

Figure 25.2 CT scan demonstrating chronic portal vein thrombosis with cavernous transformation in this patient.

• Diagnosis is usually by radiological imaging (Doppler ultrasound, CT and MRI). If the diagnosis is still uncertain formal angiography can be undertaken.

Treatment of portal vein thrombosis

• If the portal vein thrombosis is acute then aggressive attempts to recanalise the portal vein may be undertaken. This includes the use of intravenous heparin, thrombolysis and thrombectomy.

• The use of anticoagulation in the chronic setting depends on the underlying cause of the portal vein thrombosis. If there is an underlying procoagulant tendency (Box 25.1) then long-term anticoagulation is advisable after eradication of the varices. In the absence of a proven prothrombotic tendency some authorities would still recommend anticoagulation.

• TIPS is more technically challenging in the context of portal thrombosis but in expert hands the combination of either aspiration or mechanical fragmentation of the clot can be considered, followed by angioplasty before deploying a stent.

• Shunt surgery is being utilised less frequently but is considered if endoscopic therapy and radiological intervention fail to control bleeding or the subsequent complications of portal vein thrombosis.

• Portal vein thrombosis can complicate future orthotopic liver transplantation and until recently was a relative contraindication. However, by using thrombectomy, jump grafts and portal vein tributaries, there are now options for dealing with portal vein thrombosis at the time of transplantation.

Box 25.1 Examples of prothrombotic conditions in portal vein thrombosis

- Factor V Leiden mutation
- Antithombin III deficiency
- Protein C or protein S deficiency
- Myeloproliferative disorders
- Paroxysmal nocturnal haemoglobinuria
- Lupus anticoagulant syndrome

Mrs Winter is investigated for the cause of her portal vein thrombosis. There is no history of abdominal surgery, trauma or sepsis. A thrombophilia screen is requested and shows that she has protein C deficiency. Her gastric varices are eradicated by three courses of direct cyanoacrylate injection after which she is commenced on long-term anticoagulation. She continues to be seen regularly in outpatients and has no further complications.

CASE REVIEW

A 47-year-old woman presented with an emergency gastrointestinal haemorrhage. She was resuscitated and gastric varices were seen at endoscopy. There was no history of liver disease and liver function tests, including synthetic function, were normal. Investigation revealed a portal vein thrombosis without evidence of underlying liver cirrhosis. A thrombophilia screen was performed and demonstrated protein C deficiency. Her varices were eradicated by cyanoacrylate injection and she was commenced on long-term anticoagulation.

KEY POINTS

- Portal vein thrombosis can present acutely with symptoms of variceal bleeding or mesenteric ischaemia
- Liver cirrhosis may be complicated by portal vein thrombosis which can precipitate hepatic decompensation
- Imaging, with Doppler ultrasound or CT, will confirm the diagnosis. CT imaging is also useful in determining the chronicity of the thrombosis
- Treatment is directed towards the complications and aetiology of the thrombosis
- Prothrombotic tendencies need to be actively excluded in portal vein thrombosis and warrant long-term anticoagulation

Case 26 # A 37-year-old woman with abnormal liver ultrasound

Joanna Dunlop is a 37-year-old woman who is being investigated for left-sided loin pain. Her general practitioner refers her for a renal ultrasound examination which demonstrates a 7 mm calculus in the left renal pelvis. Whilst undertaking the scan the radiographer also notices an 8 cm focal lesion in her liver. She comes back to her GP to discuss the results of the scan.

What is likely to be the main concern of the patient?

She is most likely concerned that the lesion seen in her liver is cancer.

What would you tell her?

It is important to tell her that incidental lesions in the liver are very common and are usually benign. She will, however, require further investigation to ascertain the exact nature of the lesion and whether any treatment is required.

What are the causes of a focal lesion in the liver?

There are many causes of a focal abnormality within the liver. Lesions can be classified as benign or malignant. Malignant lesions may be primary (arising from liver tissue) or secondary (spread to the liver from another site, e.g. bowel, breast, lung, etc.). A list of primary malignant lesions is given in Table 26.1. Hepatocellular carcinoma and cholangiocarcinoma are the most common primary malignant lesions and are discussed in Cases 13 and 18. There are many benign causes for a focal lesion in the liver. The most important benign lesions are listed in Table 26.2.

What questions would you ask the patient?

• *Is there a history of pain?* Liver lesions do not often cause pain and in fact lesions as large as 10–15 cm are often asymptomatic. If they do cause pain it may be due to stretch of the liver capsule or to sudden haemorrhage of the lesion.

• *Is there any risk factor to suggest she might have an underlying liver disorder?* The common malignant lesions, hepatocellular carcinoma and cholangiocarcinoma, frequently develop on a background of cirrhosis or chronic biliary tract disease.

• *Is there any history of a multisystem disorder? Any other past medical history?* Some benign liver lesions are associated with multisystem disorders.

• *Is there any history of malignancy outside the liver?* This may suggest a secondary deposit in the liver.

• *Does she take any regular medication?* Some liver lesions are associated with hormonal preparations, e.g. anabolic steroids or the oral contraceptive pill.

• *Is there any family history?* Some conditions such as polycystic liver disease are familial.

• *Has there been any trauma to the abdomen?* Previous trauma with haemorrhage can sometimes result in areas of calcification in the liver.

What would you do next?

Her images need to be reviewed by an experienced radiologist. This is usually achieved by referring her case to the local hepatobiliary multidisciplinary team. Such teams usually include radiologists, pathologists, physicians, surgeons and oncologists who meet together regularly to discuss cases and decide upon appropriate investigation and treatment pathways.

She should be seen in the hepatology clinic and assessed for risk factors for liver disease, a clinical examination performed and liver function tests measured.

Table 26.1 Primary malignant neoplasms of the liver.

Tumour	Cellular origin	Notes
Hepatocellular carcinoma	Hepatocyte	Most arise on a background of cirrhosis
Cholangiocarcinoma	Biliary epithelium	Adenocarcinoma. Predisposing factors include primary sclerosing cholangitis
Angiosarcoma	Vascular endothelial cells	Cases frequently related to occupational exposure to chemicals such as vinyl chloride
Haemangioendothelioma	Vascular endothelial cells	Rare tumour, often slow growing
Biliary cystadenocarcinoma	Biliary epithelium	Malignant cystic lesions within the liver
Primary hepatic lymphoma	Lymphoid tissue	Very rare
Hepatoblastoma	Immature liver precursor cells	Rare childhood tumour

Table 26.2 Some benign lesions of the liver.

Lesion	Frequency	Notes
Cysts	Common, present in 2–5% of the population	May be single or multiple. Usually asymptomatic and no treatment is required. Occasionally can haemorrhage or cause symptoms due to their size (Fig. 26.1a)
Hydatid cyst	Uncommon in the UK and USA. Endemic in South America, New Zealand and the Mediterranean	Parasitic infection caused by tapeworms of the *Echinococcus* genus. Large complex cysts containing parasites can form in the liver, which may be asymptomatic or cause symptoms related to pressure. They may become infected or rarely rupture inducing an anaphylactic reaction to the parasites. Biopsy of hydatid cysts should be avoided as it can risk anaphylaxis
Haemangioma	Common, incidence 2-10% of the population	Cavernous vascular spaces filled with blood. Usually asymptomatic although large lesions can cause pain and may haemorrhage. Most can be diagnosed by radiological techniques (Fig. 26.1b); patients can be reassured and discharged
Focal nodular hyperplasia	Second most common benign hepatic tumour, incidence c. 0.5% of the population	Hyperplasia in response to an area of abnormal blood flow. More common in women, and may be oestrogen related. Usually asymptomatic. Diagnosed by typical radiological appearances (Fig 26.1c). Treatment rarely required
Hepatic adenoma	Uncommon	Lesions >5 cm in size have a significant risk of spontaneous haemorrhage. May be a risk of malignant transformation
Bile duct adenoma	Rare	Adenomas and cystadenomas are rare tumours that are usually asymptomatic but may cause compression of the biliary tree. Surgical resection may be required if technically feasible

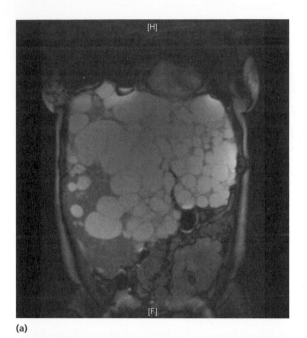

(a)

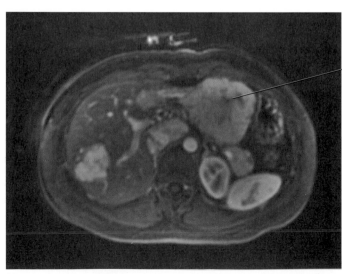

Haemangioma

(b)

Focal nodular hyperplasia
with characteristic central scar

(c)

Figure 26.1 (a) MRI scan demonstrating polycystic
liver disease. The abdomen is almost completely
filled by the polycystic liver causing pain and
discomfort for the patient. (b) MRI scan
demonstrating a liver haemangioma with
characteristic features of peripheral enhancement.
(c) MRI scan demonstrating focal nodular
hyperplasia.

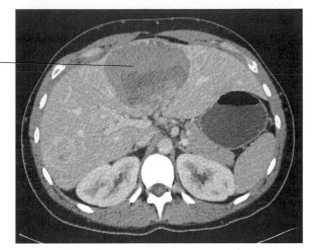

Hepatic adenoma
with haemorrhage

Figure 26.2 CT scan demonstrating a
hepatic adenoma in this patient.

*Miss Dunlop has never had any problems related to her liver
and there is no family history of liver disease. Apart from her
recent left loin pain she has never had any abdominal
symptoms. She has no past medical history but has taken
the oral contraceptive pill for 20 years. Her liver function
tests are completely normal.*

*She is referred to the hepatobiliary team who review her
images. The lesion in her liver appears solid on ultrasound,
ruling out a diagnosis of a simple cyst. She is referred for CT
examination but presents to hospital before she has the scan
with sudden onset of severe abdominal pain and
hypotension.*

*A CT scan is performed that demonstrates haemorrhage into
her liver mass (Fig. 26.2). She remains unwell with a blood
pressure that is difficult to control. She is therefore taken to
the angiography suite and undergoes emergency arterial
embolisation to control the bleeding. To prevent further
episodes she subsequently has a surgical resection removing
the area of her liver containing the liver mass. Histological
examination demonstrates a hepatic adenoma with extensive
necrosis in keeping with recent embolisation. She makes an
uneventful recovery and is discharged home.*

What do you think has happened?

Knowing that she has a large, solid, focal lesion in her
liver it is possible that she has bled into this causing her
sudden pain and fall in blood pressure. There is, however,
a wide differential diagnosis for these symptoms and
other causes such as pancreatitis, visceral perforation and
gynaecological causes, amongst others, should also be
considered.

How would you manage her?

The first priority is rapid assessment and resuscitation to
ensure that she is haemodynamically stable. Once this has
been achieved she should have emergency imaging of her
abdomen to investigate her symptoms.

CASE REVIEW

This 37-year-old woman was incidentally found to have
a large focal lesion in her liver. She was otherwise well
but had a long history of oral contraceptive use. During
the course of further investigation to characterise the
nature of the lesion she presented with symptoms suggestive of intrahepatic bleeding. This was successfully
controlled with arterial embolisation following which
she underwnent a laparotomy at which a benign hepatic
adenoma was removed.

KEY POINTS

- Focal lesions of the liver are a frequent incidental finding in an asymptomatic patient
- Benign liver lesions (e.g. cysts or haemangioma) are common and simple reassurance is usually all that is required
- Much anxiety is induced by the finding of a focal liver lesion
- Characterisation of most benign lesions can be made by radiological imaging
- Occasionally imaging gives indeterminate results and it is necessary to biopsy a benign lesion to fully characterise it
- In an asymptomatic patient with normal liver function, lesions with radiological characteristics of an individual benign tumour can usually be managed conservatively
- Embolisation or hepatic resection is rarely required for benign lesions but may be life saving in patients who develop spontaneous haemorrhage

Case 27 A 72-year-old man with right upper quadrant pain and fever

Michael Brown, a 72-year-old man, had recently been discharged from hospital following a bout of acute diverticulitis. This had been successfully managed with a course of antibiotics and he had been discharged home with his condition improving. A week later, however, he develops pain in the right upper quadrant and right shoulder tip associated with fever. He re-presents to hospital. On admission he looks unwell, has a temperature of 38.8°C and is tender in the right upper quadrant. Blood tests reveal the following:

Bilirubin	*15 μmol/L*
ALT	*87 iU/L*
ALP	*195 iU/L*
Hb	*10.8 g/dL*
WCC	*14.7 × 10⁹/L (neutrophils 11.6 × 10⁹/L)*
Plt	*480 × 10⁹/L*
CRP	*212 mg/L*

What investigations would you perform?

• *Septic screen including blood culture, urine microscopy and culture and a chest X-ray*: He is clearly unwell with a fever, raised white cell count and raised CRP. The most likely cause of this is infection. The recent history of diverticulitis and new onset of pain make an intra-abdominal source of infection likely but other causes must always be considered. He has recently been in hospital and could have a hospital-acquired infection such as chest or urinary tract infection.

• *Abdominal imaging (e.g. ultrasound or CT scan)*: His recent history of diverticulitis and these new symptoms suggest an intra-abdominal source of infection.

An ultrasound scan is performed that demonstrates normal appearance to the gallbladder and absence of biliary obstruction. There is a 5 cm lesion in the right lobe of the liver. A CT scan is performed (Fig. 27.1).

Hepatology: Clinical Cases Uncovered, 1st edition. © Kathryn Nash and Indra Neil Guha. Published 2011 by Blackwell Publishing Ltd.

What is the most likely diagnosis?

The CT scan shows a 5 cm fluid-filled lesion in the right lobe of the liver. This contains small pockets of gas and it demonstrates peripheral enhancement in the arterial phase. The most likely diagnosis is a pyogenic liver abscess.

What are the clinical features of pyogenic abscesses?

• Abdominal pain, usually localised to the right upper quadrant.
• Fever.
• Constitutional symptoms (malaise, anorexia, nausea, vomiting, weight loss).
• Diaphragmatic irritation (right shoulder tip pain, respiratory symptoms).
• Jaundice is uncommon and generally a late finding unless the abscess is causing biliary obstruction.

How can organisms get into the liver?

• Portal venous circulation (as a complication of intra-abdominal infections, e.g. appendicitis, diverticulitis, peritonitis or postoperative infections).
• Biliary tree (as a complication of cholangitis).
• Hepatic artery (as a complication of systemic bacteraemia; metastatic abscesses may be present at a number of sites within the body).
• Percutaneous (as a complication of a penetrating wound or an iatrogenic complication, e.g. following liver biopsy).

KEY POINT

• Necrotic tumours may become infected and present as a liver abscess. The possibility of an underlying neoplastic procedure should always be considered, particularly if there is no obvious predisposing factor for developing an abscess

---

155

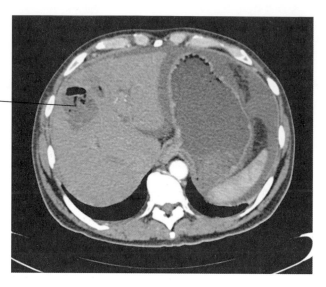

Fluid filled lesion

Figure 27.1 CT scan demonstrating a large intrahepatic abscess in this patient.

What bacteria cause hepatic abscesses?

Liver abscesses are frequently polymicrobial. Many of the causative organisms originate in the gastrointestinal tract hence enteric Gram-negative bacilli (aerobes and anaerobes) are frequently isolated:

- *Escherichia coli*
- *Klebsiella pneumonia*
- *Enterococcus* spp
- *Bacteroides* spp
- *Streptococcus* spp (milleri group and anaerobic species)
- *Proteus* spp
- *Pseudomonas* spp
- *Fusobacterium* spp.

If the infection does not originate in the gastrointestinal tract, possible organisms include:

- *Staphylococcus* spp
- *Streptococcus* spp.

What other organisms can cause liver abscesses?

- *Fungi*: Fungal abscesses are rare in immunocompetent individuals but can be seen in hepatic ischaemia or in the immunocompromised host. They are associated with a particularly poor prognosis.
- *Parasites*: Invasion of the liver by roundworms or flukes can be associated with biliary infection leading to pyogenic liver abscesses.
- *Amoeba*: The amoeba *Entamoeba histolytica* can also lead to hepatic abscesses. Cysts in contaminated food or water are ingested and release invasive trophozoites in the small intestine. These reach the colon where they invade the colonic mucosa causing amoebic dysentery. In some cases the trophozoites are carried via the portal circulation to the liver, resulting in the formation of abscesses. Clinical features and imaging findings are similar to those of bacterial abscesses. History of travel to an endemic area (e.g. India, sub-Saharan Africa or South America) may suggest the diagnosis.

What is the treatment?
Antibiotics

Antibiotics are the mainstay of treatment and should be started as soon as the diagnosis is suspected. Empirical treatment is usually given to cover enteric bacteria, including anaerobic cover (e.g. a combination of ampicillin, gentamicin and metronidazole). Microbiology advice should be sought to ascertain the local prevalence of resistant strains, particularly of *Enterobacteria*, and alternative antibiotics such as third generation cephalosporins or ampicillin/clavulonic acid or piperacillin/tazobactam combinations in place of ampicillin may be considered. Subsequent antibiotic therapy should be adjusted according to the results of bacterial cultures and sensitivity reports. Prolonged courses of antibiotics (2–6 weeks) are frequently required.

Drainage

Most abscesses will require drainage in addition to antibiotic therapy. Drainage can usually be achieved by an ultrasound or CT-guided approach, although occasionally formal surgical drainage is required. Simple aspiration of the abscess may be sufficient but frequently it is necessary to insert a drainage tube, which may need to remain in place for several days or weeks. If there are multiple abscesses, drainage of all the abscesses may not be practical and some cases are managed with antibiotics alone.

What is the prognosis?

Untreated, hepatic abscesses have a very poor prognosis with near 100% mortality. The combination of needle aspiration and antibiotic therapy has reduced mortality to 10–25%. Poor prognosis is associated with multiple liver abscesses, old age, coexisting medical conditions and jaundice.

The liver abscess is drained under ultrasound guidance revealing thick purulent fluid which grows Escherichia coli. Mr Brown is started on intravenous ampicillin, gentamicin and metronidazole therapy, which results in improvement in his inflammatory markers. He has a repeat ultrasound after 2 weeks of therapy that demonstrates that the abscess cavity is significantly reduced in size. He is due to be changed to oral antibiotics and discharged home but he suddenly develops watery diarrhoea with his bowels opening six times a day.

What is the most likely cause of his diarrhoea?

The most probable cause is antibiotic-associated diarrhoea.

What other causes of diarrhoea should be considered?

• *Diverticular disease*: His initial problem was caused by diverticulitis. The return of diarrhoea could herald an exacerbation of this chronic condition.
• *Colorectal neoplasm*: Colorectal cancer with metastatic disease should be considered as an underlying cause in any case presenting with liver abscesses.

What is the mechanism of antibiotic-associated diarrhoea?

Antibiotics disturb the balance of the normal gastrointestinal bacteria and can lead to a proliferation of harmful bacteria that can produce diarrhoea. This is a common side effect of antibiotic therapy and often resolves as soon as the antibiotics are discontinued and the normal microbial species are re-established.

The most serious form of antibiotic-associated diarrhoea is overpopulation with the anaerobic, Gram-positive, spore-forming bacillus *Clostridium difficile*. This bacterium is present in the hospital environment where it can persist in spore form. Infection is spread by the faecal–oral route. Overgrowth of *C. difficile* in the gastrointestinal tract and release of toxins A and B results in diarrhoea, bloating and in its most severe form inflammation and ulceration of the colonic mucosa with the development of pseudomembranes (pseudomembranous colitis).

How is *C. difficile*-associated diarrhoea diagnosed?

Diagnosis is made by detecting the bacterial toxin in the stool of a symptomatic patient. Detecting the presence of the bacteria alone is not sufficient to diagnose *C. difficile*-associated diarrhoea since it is a normal commensal organism in the bowel in many individuals.

How do you treat *C. difficile*-associated diarrhoea?

Metronidazole or vancomycin are the main antibiotics used to treat *C. difficile* diarrhoea. Metronidazole is the drug of choice as it is less expensive and has comparable efficacy with vancomycin. Treatment course is usually for 10–14 days although some patients relapse when treatment is discontinued.

Why did he develop *C. difficile* diarrhoea if he was already on metronidazole?

• Some strains of *C. difficile* are resistant to metronidazole.
• He was on intravenous metronidazole which does not give high concentrations of antibiotic in the gut lumen where the bacteria are located.

KEY POINT

• Treatment for *C. difficile* diarrhoea should be with oral antibiotics to ensure that the drug gets to the site of infection

What other precautions should be undertaken in managing patients with *C. difficile* diarrhoea?

Patients should be nursed in isolation in a side room with its own toilet facilities to minimise the spread of infection to other patients. Staff and visitors should wear gloves and aprons when interacting with the patient and wash their hands with soap and water after each encounter.

KEY POINT

- The spores of *C. difficile* are not destroyed by alcohol gel. When caring for patients with known or suspected *C. difficile* diarrhoea, hand washing should be undertaken with soap and water

Stool samples are sent and test positive for C. difficile toxin. In view of his recent treatment with metronidazole and the possibility that his strain of C. difficile is resistant to that antibiotic, he is commenced on oral vancomycin. His diarrhoea settles down over the next 5 days and he is discharged home to complete a 2-week course of treatment.

CASE REVIEW

This 72-year-old man presented with abdominal pain, fever and deranged liver function tests shortly after a bout of diverticulitis. Radiological imaging demonstrated a liver abscess which was treated with a combination of aspiration and antibiotics. He subsequently developed an episode of *C. difficile* diarrhoea which resolved with a course of oral vancomycin.

KEY POINTS

- Liver abscesses usually present with constitutional upset, abdominal pain and fever
- Most infections originate in the biliary tree or the abdomen via portal venous spread, although some abscesses complicate systemic spread via the hepatic artery
- Infection is frequently polymicrobial and caused by bacteria of the gastrointestinal tract
- Management usually requires a combination of radiological aspiration and prolonged courses of antibiotics
- Broad spectrum antibiotic usage can lead to overgrowth of bacteria such as *C. difficile* in the gastrointestinal tract resulting in diarrhoea
- Treatment for *C. difficile* diarrhoea is with oral metronidazole or vancomycin

A 52-year-old man with diarrhoea and a liver mass

Roy Perkins is a 52-year-old man who presents with a 6-month history of abdominal pain and diarrhoea. His bowels are opening up to five times a day with a loose watery stool but no blood. He has lost 5 kg in weight. His only past medical history is an appendicectomy 8 years previously. At the time he was told that his appendix contained a 4 cm tumour but he is unable to recall the details.

On examination he has an enlarged liver extending 6 cm below the right costal margin. He also appears to have a flushed, red face. He reports that this flushing has been present for the past few months; it typically increases in intensity following meals or alcohol and can be associated with wheezing. An urgent colonoscopy examination is performed which is normal, but CT examination of the abdomen demonstrates several lesions within the liver (Fig. 28.1).

What is the likely diagnosis?

The symptoms of diarrhoea with facial flushing in a patient with multiple liver lesions strongly suggest the carcinoid syndrome.

What is the primary tumour? Where does it arise?

Carcinoid tumours are neoplasms arising from the neuroendocrine system. Most primary tumours arise from the gastrointestinal tract and may be classified depending on their point of origin as foregut (stomach and duodenum), midgut (ileum and proximal colon) or hindgut (distal colon and rectum). Midgut tumours are the most common; they are frequently asymptomatic but may present as bowel obstruction or as an incidental finding following appendicectomy for acute appendicitis. Other rare sites of origin of carcinoid tumours include the lungs and thymus gland.

Hepatology: Clinical Cases Uncovered, 1st edition. © Kathryn Nash and Indra Neil Guha. Published 2011 by Blackwell Publishing Ltd.

Mr Perkins most likely had an appendiceal primary that was resected when he presented with acute appendicitis 8 years previously. Most appendiceal tumours are relatively benign and are cured by appendicectomy. A few cases, particularly those with tumours >2 cm, develop secondary spread and present several years later with metastatic disease.

What is the natural history of the primary tumour?

Primary carcinoid tumours are typically slow growing and can be present for many years before they cause symptoms. When they do present it is often with bowel obstruction.

What is the cause of his current symptoms?

Carcinoid tumours produce a number of hormones including serotonin, also known as 5-hydroxytryptamine (5-HT). If 5-HT reaches the systemic circulation it can produce the symptoms of flushing, bronchospasm and diarrhoea. Primary gut carcinoid tumours secrete 5-HT into the portal circulation; it passes to the liver and is inactivated there. Thus, the carcinoid syndrome is not present when tumours are confined to the gastrointestinal primary site. In the presence of liver metastases, 5-HT is secreted directly into the systemic circulation and the patient may develop symptoms.

What cardiac abnormalities may occur?

Serotonin may induce fibrosis of the tricuspid and pulmonary valves resulting in stenosis or valvular insufficiency.

What test would you perform to make the diagnosis?

5-HT is broken down to 5-hydroxyindoleacetic acid (5-HIAA), which is excreted in the urine. A 24-hour urine collection should be performed; an elevated urinary

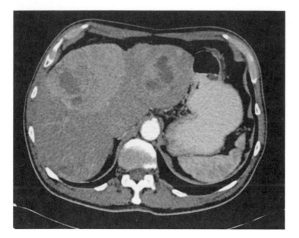

Figure 28.1 CT scan demonstrating multiple lesions within the liver in this patient.

5-HIAA level is characteristic of the carcinoid syndrome.

If the primary site is unknown what test could help to identify it?

The primary site is often not visible on CT or MRI imaging. An octreotide scan may help in localising the primary tumour. Carcinoid tumour cells frequently have receptors for somatostatin. Octreotide is a synthetic somatostatin analogue. Radioactive indium-111-labelled octreotide given to the patient can bind to the somatostatin receptors on the carcinoid tumour and appear as bright areas on an octreotide scan. This test is used in the detection of liver metastases and localisation of the primary tumour.

What options are available for treatment?

• *Surgery*: If complete surgical resection is possible then the patient could be considered for this radical approach. Frequently, however, the metastases are too extensive for this to be feasible. Liver transplantation has been performed in carefully selected patients.

• *Hepatic embolisation*: Liver metastases are highly vascular and respond well to radiological embolisation of their blood supply. A catheter is inserted into the femoral artery and under fluoroscopic guidance is passed into the hepatic artery where the tumour vessels can be identified and blocked. Some patients require multiple embolisations over many years to control symptoms.

• *Pharmacological treatment*: Octreotide is effective in controlling symptoms of the carcinoid syndrome, particularly flushing and diarrhoea. The disadvantage is that it has to be given subcutaneously and has a short half-life so has to be given multiple times a day. Slow release formulations are now available.

• *Cytotoxic chemotherapy*: Most agents produce disappointing results and this treatment should only be considered as a last resort when embolisation and pharmacological treatment have failed.

Mr Perkins is started on octreotide injections which control his symptoms. It is felt that his liver disease is too extensive for surgical resection and he undergoes hepatic embolisation with reduction in the tumour load in his liver.

CASE REVIEW

This man had an appendicectomy at which time an appendiceal tumour was resected. He was unable to recall the details but his presentation several years later with flushing, diarrhoea and wheeze strongly suggested metastatic neuroendocrine tumour with the carcinoid syndrome. His liver contained many secondary deposits such that curative surgery was not possible. His symptoms were controlled with the somatostatin analogue, octreotide, and the tumour mass was reduced by hepatic embolisation.

KEY POINTS

• Carcinoid tumours are rare neoplasms of the neuroendocrine system, most frequently originating in the midgut
• The primary tumours progress slowly and are frequently asymptomatic for many years
• Development of the carcinoid syndrome implies metastatic spread to the liver and secretion of 5-HT into the systemic circulation
• An elevated 24-hour urine 5-HIAA is suggestive of the carcinoid syndrome
• Treatment options for symptoms of the carcinoid syndrome include surgical resection or embolisation of hepatic lesions or octreotide pharmacotherapy

A 69-year-old man with a liver mass

PART 2: CASES

Bill Jones is a 69-year-old man who underwent a right hemicolectomy for adenocarcinoma of the ascending colon. Histological examination of the resected tumour demonstrated that the cancer had invaded through the bowel wall and half of the resected lymph nodes contained tumour deposits making it a Dukes' C carcinoma. Following recovery from his surgery he received a 6-month course of chemotherapy which he tolerated well and a CT scan a year after the initial diagnosis showed no sign of tumour recurrence.

Two years following completion of his chemotherapy he is reviewed in the clinic and found to have a palpable liver. A CT scan is organised that demonstrates a solitary 6cm lesion in the right lobe of the liver (Fig. 29.1).

What is the most likely diagnosis?

Metastatic colorectal carcinoma.

What investigations may be undertaken to confirm the diagnosis?

A patient with typical appearances of liver metastases and a recent history of colorectal carcinoma may not require any further investigation. Benign lesions of the liver are, however, common and if there is any doubt as to the nature of a liver lesion then further investigation will be required:

• Many colorectal carcinomas produce the tumour marker carcinoembryonic antigen (CEA). It is not specific for the disorder but can be helpful in detecting recurrence in patients where elevated CEA levels return to normal after treatment of the primary tumour.

• Positron emission tomography (PET) scanning may be helpful in demonstrating recurrence and in determining whether a lesion in the liver is malignant or not. Radioactive fluorodeoxyglucose ([18]FDG) is taken up in

cancerous tissues, which are seen as spots on a scan. Colon cancer is an [18]FDG-avid disease and usually shows up on PET imaging.

• If curative treatment is possible, many centres will not perform a percutaneous biopsy of the liver lesions due to the risk of tumour seedlings spreading down the needle track.

> **!RED FLAG**
>
> Potentially resectable colorectal liver metastases should not be biopsied without discussing the case with a liver surgical centre.

What other investigations should be performed?

• It is important to investigate whether the cancer has spread anywhere else. If a whole body PET scan has not been undertaken it is important to image the chest, usually with a CT scan.

• A colonoscopy should be performed if he has not had one in the last year to exclude a second colorectal primary tumour.

What treatment options are available?

• *Surgical resection of liver metastases*: Liver resection may be curative, although patients are frequently not fit enough for this complex procedure and the number, location and size of the metastases may mean that resection is not technically possible. The average 5-year survival following liver resection for colorectal metastases is 25–30%; the outlook is better if there is a solitary lesion.

• *Radiofrequency ablation (RFA)*: RFA uses heat to destroy cancer cells in the liver. It involves placing electrodes into the tumour under ultrasound guidance. The electrodes are used to heat the tumour with the aim of destroying it. RFA can be applied percutaneously or during surgery.

Hepatology: Clinical Cases Uncovered, 1st edition. © Kathryn Nash and Indra Neil Guha. Published 2011 by Blackwell Publishing Ltd.

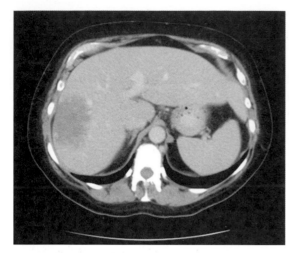

Figure 29.1 CT scan of this patient.

Box 29.1 Factors that impair the ability of the liver to regenerate

- Increasing age
- Cirrhosis or advanced fibrosis
- Steatosis
- Hepatitis
- Preoperative chemotherapy
- Ischaemia

• *Chemotherapy*: Chemotherapy may be used as an adjunct to surgical or radiological approaches or may be used alone, when its use would be considered to prolong life rather than aiming to cure the disease.

> *Mr Jones undergoes a colonoscopy which is normal and a PET scan which shows no evidence of disease outside of the liver. His CEA is elevated, having been normal 6 months previously. His images are reviewed by radiologists and hepatobiliary surgeons and it is felt that he is a candidate for surgical resection.*

What factors need to be considered when contemplating hepatic resection?

• *Fitness for the operation*: Liver resection is a major procedure with an operative mortality of 3–8%. An anaesthetic assessment is essential to determine the patient's fitness for the procedure. Recently, laparoscopic liver resections have been performed that may reduce morbidity and mortality.

• *Number and location of tumour deposits*: The location of the tumour deposits is a key determinant of whether surgical resection is technically feasible. Detailed radiological assessment is necessary to determine the precise location of the tumour deposits and their relationships to the hepatic vasculature. Deposits confined to one lobe may be removed by a lobectomy. If there is bilobar disease it is frequently not possible to undertake a curative resection although it may sometimes be possible to perform a lobectomy and also perform small wedge excisions of peripheral deposits in the other lobe.

• *Size of the liver resection*: The liver is remarkable in its ability to regenerate and it is this phenomenon that makes major liver surgery possible. It is important, however, to ensure that sufficient tissue remains to provide essential hepatic functions whilst the liver is undertaking this period of regeneration. Generally resection of 50% of the liver is well tolerated without major morbidity, and in a carefully selected cases resection of 60–70% of the liver may be tolerated.

• *State of the background liver*: The ability of the liver to regenerate is determined by the state of the background hepatic tissue. The factors that impair liver regeneration are given in Box 29.1. If any of these factors are present patients are less able to tolerate major hepatic resection.

• *Extrahepatic disease*: Whether there is extrahepatic metastatic disease needs to be determined by CT or PET examination. The presence of such disease is not necessarily a contraindication to undertaking hepatic resection since radiological approaches for treating metastatic deposits and even lung surgery can be undertaken in carefully selected cases.

What are the complications of hepatic resection?

• *Bleeding*: During liver surgery several major vascular structures are divided and can cause bleeding. In addition, the liver is a highly vascular organ and bleeding from the cut edge of the remnant liver may occur.

• *Infection*: Any surgical procedure can predispose to infection (e.g. wound, urinary tract, pneumonia). If there is hepatic dysfunction the ability to prevent and respond to infection is impaired, resulting in an increased risk and increased severity of clinical infective episodes.

• *Hepatic failure*: Insufficient liver mass to undertake essential hepatic functions leads to liver failure. This may be manifest by coagulopathy, infection, renal dysfunction and encephalopathy and may result in death.

• *Bile leak*: Leakage of bile from the cut surface of the liver or the divided bile ducts can occur. Bile is a chemical irritant and leakage into the abdomen causes pain and inflammation and acts as a nidus for infection.

• *Fluid collections*: Following liver surgery, fluid may collect in the abdomen as ascites or discrete collections, e.g. in the subphrenic space. Such collections may become infected, requiring radiological or surgical drainage. In addition, surgery close to the diaphragm can result in pleural irritation with the development of a pleural effusion.

• *Other surgical complications*: He is at risk of other surgical complications including thromboembolic disease, wound leaks and pulmonary atelectasis.

Mr Jones is reviewed by an anaesthetist and is felt to be fit for liver surgery. He undergoes a right hemihepatectomy and makes an uncomplicated postoperative recovery. Histology of the resected specimen confirms metastatic adenocarcinoma.

CASE REVIEW

Mr Jones had a history of colorectal primary cancer which had been treated with surgical resection and chemotherapy. Two years later he was found to have a palpable liver and CT examination demonstrated a solitary lesion in the right lobe of the liver consistent with a metastatic deposit. He underwent a liver resection which he tolerated well and was discharged home.

KEY POINTS

• The most frequently encountered liver tumour is one that is metastatic
• Venous drainage of the gastrointestinal tract into the portal vein results in metastatic spread of colorectal carcinoma to the liver
• Treatment options for colorectal hepatic metastases include liver resection, radiofrequency ablation and chemotherapy

• Liver resection is performed with curative intent; 5-year survival is in the order of 25–50%
• Liver resection is a major undertaking. Prior to performing the procedure it is vital to assess the patient's overall fitness, the distribution of their disease and the ability of their background liver to regenerate

Case 30 A 56-year-old man with abnormal liver function tests 4 weeks after liver transplantation

Martin Young is a 56-year-old man who underwent liver transplantation. He was discharged home 3 weeks after his transplant with normal liver function tests. At his outpatient visit a week later he is feeling well but his liver function tests are noted to be abnormal:

Bilirubin	*42 µmol/L*
ALT	*279 iU/L*
ALP	*163 iU/L*
CRP	*68 mg/L*

What questions would you ask him?

• *What was the indication for liver transplantation?* The indication for liver transplantation may have a bearing on the risk of certain complications following transplantation. For example, patients with autoimmune disease may be more likely to get rejection; those with a biliary aetiology may be more likely to get a biliary complication. Indications for liver transplantation are given in Box 30.1 and contraindications in Box 30.2.

• *Has he had a fever?* A fever might suggest infection. Further questions should be asked, for example does he have respiratory or urinary symptoms, redness or discharge from his wound?

• *Is there any pain?* It is common to have some pain following a transplant but it should be improving by week 4 and controlled by simple analgesia.

• *Any other symptoms (e.g. nausea, vomiting, bowel disturbance)?*

• *What medication is he taking?*

What other information might be helpful?

• *Operation details:* The operation note should be examined as there may be special surgical considerations that

need to be taken into account in his presentation. The patient himself is unlikely to be aware of these details.

• *Postoperative course:* Again, the patient himself may not be aware of the details of any early postoperative issues, therefore the notes should be examined carefully.

Mr Young had his transplant for cirrhosis secondary to hepatitic C. The operation itself was relatively straightforward. Three days following the operation he was diagnosed with a postoperative chest infection that responded well to antibiotics. Otherwise his postoperative course was uncomplicated and he was discharged home on three immunosuppressive drugs, tacrolimus, azathioprine and prednisolone. Since he has been home he has felt well in himself, he has not had a fever and his pain has been manageable on paracetamol and occasional opiate analgesia. On examination he looks well but is mildly jaundiced. His temperature is 37.8°C. His heart sounds are normal and his chest is clear. His abdominal wound appears to be healing well and is only slightly tender. There is no organomegaly and no free fluid evident in his abdomen.

What complications should be considered in this early post-transplant period?

• *Infection:* Post-transplant infection is common with bacterial infection predominating (Box 30.3). CMV is a particular risk if a CMV-positive donor is used for a CMV-negative recipient. Other viral infections are rarely a problem. Local fungal infections are common and can be treated with topical therapy. Systemic fungal infection is fortunately rare, usually occurring in hospitalised patients who are already ill.

• Rejection.

• Surgical complications (Box 30.4).

• Recurrent disease: This rarely causes a problem in the first few weeks but is a significant concern in the long term.

Hepatology: Clinical Cases Uncovered, 1st edition. © Kathryn Nash and Indra Neil Guha. Published 2011 by Blackwell Publishing Ltd.

> **Box 30.1 Indications for liver transplantation**
>
> - Cirrhosis with complications, for example:
>   - poor synthetic function
>   - complicated ascites (e.g. diuretic-resistant ascites or episodes of spontaneous bacterial peritonitis)
>   - encephalopathy
>   - others (e.g. pulmonary disease)
> - Acute liver failure: paracetamol and non-paracetamol aetiology
> - Hepatocellular carcinoma: selected patients according to size and number of tumours
> - Others, for example:
>   - failed liver transplant (e.g. hepatic artery thrombosis, chronic rejection, disease recurrence)
>   - inherited metabolic disorders
>   - polycystic liver disease
>   - intractable itch in primary biliary cirrhosis

> **Box 30.2 Contraindications for liver transplantation**
>
> - Acquired immune deficiency syndrome
> - Cholangiocarcinoma
> - Infection outside the hepatobiliary system
> - Active alcohol or substance abuse
> - Malignancy outside the liver (not skin cancer)
> - Advanced co-morbidity (e.g. advanced heart, lung or neurological condition)
> - Diffuse venous thrombosis (portal and mesenteric venous system)

> **Box 30.3 Examples of common infections seen in the early post-transplant course**
>
> - Bacterial:
>   - chest (pneumonia, empyema)
>   - urine
>   - wound
>   - intra-abdominal collection
>   - gastrointestinal (e.g. *Clostridium difficile* diarrhoea)
> - Viral: cytomegalovirus
> - Fungal: *Candida* (e.g. oral thrush)

What investigations would you recommend?

- *Septic screen*:
  - Blood cultures
  - Urine culture

> **Box 30.4 Surgical complications after liver transplantation**
>
> - Bleeding (usually occurs at the time of transplantation or in the first few days)
> - Vascular:
>   - hepatic artery thrombosis
>   - portal vein thrombosis
>   - vena cava obstruction/stenosis
> - Biliary:
>   - leaks
>   - strictures

  - Wound swab
  - Chest X-ray.
- *Abdominal ultrasound*:
  - Assess liver texture
  - Doppler examination to assess vessel patency
  - Exclude biliary dilatation that might suggest a bile duct stricture
  - Examine for intra-abdominal collections that could indicate a source of infection or a complication such as a bile leak.
- *Consider a liver biopsy*: If there is no obvious sepsis or surgical complication to account for the deranged liver function tests, patients may require a liver biopsy to investigate post-transplant abnormal liver function tests

An algorithm for the investigation of abnormal liver function tests following liver transplantation is given in Fig. 30.1.

There is no evidence of sepsis and liver ultrasound examination demonstrates patent vessels, no biliary duct dilatation and no intra-abdominal collections. A liver biopsy is performed that demonstrates a mixed inflammatory cell infiltrate and endothelialitis characteristic of acute cellular rejection.

What types of rejection do you know?

- *Hyperacute rejection*: This occurs immediately due to preformed antibodies, e.g. ABO incompatibility. Patients undergoing liver transplantation are matched for blood group and this form of rejection is not seen.
- *Acute cellular rejection*: This is common, probably occurring in over 50% of transplants although not all episodes are symptomatic. It occurs early in the first few weeks post-transplantation due to T-cell recognition of HLA mismatches. It is characterised by deterioration in liver blood tests and may be accompanied by a fever.

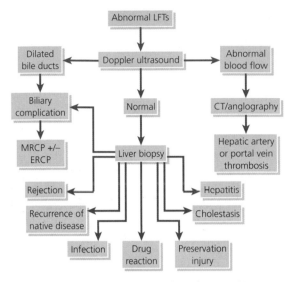

Figure 30.1 Algorithm for the investigation of abnormal liver function tests following liver transplantation.

Mild episodes may settle spontaneously although more severe episodes will require treatment with high doses of corticosteroids.

• *Chronic ductopenic rejection*: This is less common, affecting 3–7% of transplants. It occurs later with a peak onset at 3 months. The presentation is with jaundice, itching, elevated alkaline phosphatase and histology showing a paucity of bile ducts within portal tracts. No medical treatment is of proven benefit and patients may require a second transplant.

Mr Young receives high dose immunosuppression with three pulses of methylprednisolone and his liver function tests promptly settle and he is discharged home. He continues to improve and is well when seen in the outpatient clinic a year later.

What is his prognosis now?

The long-term outlook for patients who undergo liver transplantation is excellent. One-year survival following liver transplantation is just over 90% and 5-year survival approaches 80%.

What are the main long-term complications of liver transplantation?
Complications of immunosuppression

• *Infection*: The risk of infection is highest in the early post-transplant period but patients remain at risk and should be advised to seek attention if there are any symp-

toms or signs of infection. They should be reminded to have vaccinations for influenza each year.

• *Vascular disease*: Immunosuppressant drugs are complicated by diabetes, hypertension and weight gain, which increase the risk of vascular disease. Patients should be assessed for this risk and treated accordingly.

• *Renal impairment*: Tacrolimus, and the other commonly used primary immunosuppressant drug ciclosporin, are nephrotoxic and renal impairment is common with long-term use.

• *Malignancy*: Immunosuppression increases the risk of malignancy. Patients should be advised to wear sun cream and should have appropriate screening, e.g. cervical smears. Transplantation can be complicated by lymphoproliferation when it is known as post-transplant lymphoproliferative disorder.

Disease recurrence

One of the greatest threats to long-term graft outlook is disease recurrence, especially viral hepatitis, but also autoimmune disease, fatty liver disease and use of alcohol.

CASE REVIEW

A 56-year-old man developed abnormal liver function tests 4 weeks after having a relatively uncomplicated liver transplant for hepatitis C-related cirrhosis. On examination there was no evidence of infection. Blood and fluid cultures were negative and a liver ultrasound was normal. He underwent a liver biopsy that demonstrated acute cellular rejection. He was treated with corticosteroids and made a good recovery.

KEY POINTS

• Liver transplantation is indicated for carefully selected patients with end-stage liver disease, acute liver failure and some patients with hepatocellular carcinoma
• Early complications include infection, rejection and post-surgical complications
• Acute rejection is common but most cases settle with corticosteroids
• Chronic rejection is less common but no effective therapy exists and patients frequently need re-transplantation
• Long-term complications include disease recurrence and complications related to the side effects of immunosuppression

MCQs

For each question below select the single best answer.

1 *A 42-year-old woman presents with right upper quadrant pain and jaundice associated with pale stools and dark urine. On direct questioning she admits that she has had recurrent bouts of pain over the past year. These usually occur after fatty meals, last for several hours and are associated with nausea and vomiting.*

Which one of the following statements is likely to be correct?
a. The most likely diagnosis is carcinoma of the head of the pancreas
b. The gallbladder is likely to be palpable
c. The dark urine is due to the presence of excess urobilinogen
d. A prolonged prothrombin time indicates that she is developing liver failure
e. The most appropriate first-line test is an abdominal ultrasound

2 *A 2-week-old infant is investigated because of mild jaundice. He was born at term with a normal birth weight. He is breast fed and is otherwise well and is putting on weight. Jaundice developed on the second day of life. His urine and stools are a normal colour.*

What is the most likely cause of his jaundice?
a. Biliary atresia
b. Neonatal cytomegalovirus infection
c. Crigler–Najjar syndrome
d. Physiological 'breast milk' jaundice
e. Hypothyroidism

3 *A 41-year-old man with a long history of excess alcohol intake and known oesophageal varices presents to the emergency department having vomited a large amount of blood. He is pale and clammy with a pulse of 110 beats per minute and BP of 85/60 mmHg.*

Which one of the following statements is true?
a. The immediate priority is to undertake upper gastrointestinal endoscopy to control the bleeding
b. He has a 70% risk of dying on this admission
c. It is important to administer broad spectrum antibiotics as soon as possible
d. Terlipressin reduces portal pressure by causing splanchnic arteriolar vasodilatation
e. The best endoscopic treatment is to inject varices with adrenaline

4 *A 34-year-old man consults his GP as he has noticed himself to be jaundiced. He has been unwell for the past week with a flu-like illness. There is no abdominal pain and his urine and stools are a normal colour. Investigation reveals an elevated bilirubin but the rest of his liver function tests are normal.*

What is the most likely diagnosis?
a. Hepatitis A infection
b. EBV infection (glandular fever)
c. Gilbert's syndrome
d. Cirrhosis
e. Overdosing of paracetamol for his flu-like illness

Hepatology: Clinical Cases Uncovered, 1st edition. © Kathryn Nash and Indra Neil Guha. Published 2011 by Blackwell Publishing Ltd.

PART 3: SELF-ASSESSMENT

5 *A 23-year-old woman from Pakistan is found to be a chronic carrier of hepatitis B virus. She has normal liver function tests, is HBeAg positive, anti-HBe negative and has a high level of HBV DNA in her blood.*

Which one of the following statements is true?
a. She requires lifelong treatment to suppress viral replication
b. She has normal liver function tests and is therefore not an infection risk to others
c. She most likely acquired the infection at birth or in early childhood
d. As her liver function tests are normal she does not require further follow-up
e. She will have a positive test for IgM anti-HBc antibody

6 *A 33-year-old woman is investigated for right upper quadrant pain and undergoes ultrasound examination. Gallstones are seen in her gallbladder but in addition she is found to have a 3 cm lesion on her liver. She has taken the oral contraceptive pill for 10 years.*

Which one of the following statements is true?
a. The lesion is likely to be malignant and she should have an urgent CT scan
b. The lesion in her liver is probably the cause of her pain
c. The lesion should be biopsied to establish a diagnosis
d. The oral contraceptive pill can be safely continued
e. Her ultrasound should be reviewed by the hepatobiliary multidisciplinary team to decide on further management

7 *A 53-year-old man with known haemochromatosis and cirrhosis is seen in the liver clinic. He is asymptomatic but has a strong family history of hepatocellular carcinoma (HCC) in that both his father and brother died of the disorder.*

Regarding investigation for HCC, which of the following statements is true?
a. A normal α-fetoprotein excludes the diagnosis
b. The CT finding of arterial enhancement of a lesion followed by washout in the portal venous phase are suggestive of a diagnosis of HCC
c. Histology is mandatory to diagnose HCC
d. Ultrasound is not a useful screening tool for HCC in cirrhosis as it cannot differentiate a malignant lesion from the background nodular liver
e. HCC is frequently symptomatic therefore investigation should be reserved for those who present with symptoms

8 *A 66-year-old man with a long history of ulcerative colitis treated with azathioprine is found to have abnormal liver function tests. His bilirubin and ALT are normal but alkaline phosphatase is three times the upper limit of normal.*

What is the most likely diagnosis?
a. Primary sclerosing cholangitis
b. Primary biliary cirrhosis
c. Autoimmune hepatitis
d. Azathioprine hepatotoxicity
e. Colorectal cancer with hepatic metastases

9 *A 21-year-old man consults his GP with a 2-week history of lethargy, nausea and myalgia. For the last 2 days he has had generalised discomfort in his upper abdomen and he has noticed that his urine is dark in colour. Blood tests demonstrate that his bilirubin is slightly elevated, as is his alkaline phosphatase, but his ALT is over 2000 iU/L.*

What is the most likely diagnosis?
a. Wilson's disease
b. Acute viral hepatitis
c. Gallstone obstruction of the common bile duct
d. Gilbert's syndrome
e. Acute alcoholic hepatitis

10 *An 83-year-old man is found to have abnormal liver function tests. He was admitted 3 days previously having lost consciousness at home. When the paramedics found him he was hypotensive with a blood pressure of 75/50 mmHg. He had ECG changes consistent with a myocardial infarction, his troponin was elevated and he had signs of cardiac failure. With treatment his clinical condition improved but his liver function tests became abnormal: bilirubin 85 μmol/L, ALT 1936 iU/L, alkaline phosphatase 172 iU/L.*

What is the most likely diagnosis?
a. Acute viral hepatitis
b. Drug reaction
c. Budd–Chiari syndrome
d. Haemochromatosis
e. Ischaemic hepatitis

11 *A 25-year-old woman presents to the emergency department having taken a large overdose of paracetamol 36 hours previously.*

Which of the following statements is true?
a. Renal failure is a rare complication of paracetamol overdose
b. *N*-acetyl cysteine is of no benefit if started more than 16 hours after the overdose
c. The degree of elevation of the ALT at this stage is important in determining her prognosis
d. If she is taking antiepileptic drugs she should be treated with *N*-acetyl cysteine at lower serum levels of paracetamol than patients who do not take these agents
e. If her INR is elevated it should be corrected immediately with vitamin K and fresh frozen plasma

12 *A 36-week pregnant woman mentions to her midwife that she has been itching. It began when she was 34 weeks pregnant and initially affected her legs and feet but now she has generalised pruritus. Blood tests are taken that demonstrate a normal bilirubin but a raised ALT and alkaline phosphatase. Her full blood count was normal and a liver ultrasound unremarkable. She has never had any problems with her liver before and is otherwise fit and well and has no abdominal pain.*

What is the most likely diagnosis?
a. Intrahepatic cholestasis of pregnancy
b. Hepatitis C virus infection
c. Acute fatty liver of pregnancy
d. HELLP syndrome
e. Primary biliary cirrhosis

13 *A 65-year-old man is referred to the hepatology clinic because he has been found to have a raised ALT of 110 iU/L. On examination he has a tanned complexion and a slim build with a body mass index of 22 kg/m². He was diagnosed with diabetes 2 years previously and also suffers from atrial fibrillation for which he takes warfarin and digoxin. His only other medication is occasional paracetamol for painful wrists and knees.*

What is the most likely cause of his raised ALT?
a. Drug-induced liver injury
b. Wilson's disease
c. Hereditary haemochromatosis
d. Cardiac congestion
e. Alpha-1 antitrypsin deficiency

14 *A 15-year-old boy is referred to the liver clinic with ataxia and abnormal liver function tests. His hepatologist considers a diagnosis of Wilson's diesase.*

Which of the following statements is true?
a. A normal serum caeruloplasmin excludes Wilson's disease
b. The presence of Kayser–Fleischer rings is diagnostic of Wilson's disease
c. The diagnosis of Wilson's disease is unlikely as patients classically present with liver disease in middle age
d. Penicillamine is often used to treat Wilson's disease
e. Neurological symptoms of Wilson's disease usually get better once treatment is commenced

15 *A 72-year-old man who is under the haematologists for polycythaemia rubra vera presents to the emergency department with a 2-day history of abdominal pain. On examination he is mildly jaundiced and there are no signs of chronic liver disease but he has a painful enlarged liver with moderate ascites.*

What is the most likely diagnosis?
a. Malignant infiltration of the liver
b. Acute alcoholic hepatitis
c. Budd–Chiari syndrome
d. Hepatitis A virus infection
e. Acute autoimmune hepatitis

16 *A 58-year-old man with longstanding primary sclerosing cholangitis (PSC) and cirrhosis comes to clinic early because he has developed jaundice. Ultrasound examination demonstrates bile duct dilatation in the left lobe of the liver, there are no gallstones and no mass lesion is seen.*

Which one of the following statements is true?
a. An elevated CA19.9 in this setting would be diagnostic of cholangiocarcinoma
b. As there is no mass seen on ultrasound he should be started on ursodeoxycholic acid and reassured
c. In the absence of gallstones the cause of his jaundice will be a malignant complication of primary sclerosing cholangitis
d. Further investigation should include a MRCP and CT scan
e. If he has developed cholangiocarcinoma, liver transplantation should be considered

17 *A 24-year-old woman is referred to the liver clinic as she has been found to be hepatitis C virus positive.*

Regarding risk factors for acquiring hepatitis C virus, which of the following statements is true?
a. Heterosexual sexual exposure is rarely associated with transmitting the virus
b. If she was an intravenous drug user but has never shared needles it is unlikely that she acquired the virus via this route
c. HCV is transmitted very efficiently transplacentally and over 90% of children born to RNA positive mothers acquire the virus

d. Following a needlestick injury from an HCV-positive patient the risk of transmission of HCV is about 90%
e. HCV RNA positive mothers should not breast feed to reduce the risk of transmitting the virus to the neonate

18 *A 58-year-old woman with abnormal liver function tests is seen in the liver clinic and referred for a liver biopsy.*

Which of the following statements is true:
a. Liver biopsy can be safely performed by the percutaneous route in a patient with an INR of 2
b. In a patient with ascites it is preferred to perform a liver biopsy via the transjugular route
c. The incidence of fatal haemorrhage from percutaneous liver biopsy is 1%
d. Patients with bile duct obstruction can safely undergo liver biopsy by the transjugular route
e. All cystic lesions in the liver should be biopsied to confirm their aetiology

19 *A 35-year-old doctor receives a needle stick injury from a HCV-positive patient on the hepatology ward.*

Regarding hepatitis C virus infection, which of the following statements is true?
a. Most people who acquire the virus develop jaundice associated with clearance of the virus from the blood
b. Over 90% of chronic carriers of the virus will eventually develop cirrhosis
c. Response to antiviral therapy and clearance of the virus results in loss of HCV RNA and HCV antibody from the serum
d. Current treatment regimens for HCV are associated with approximately a 50% chance of eradicating the virus
e. Patients with HCV infection are not eligible for liver transplantation as there is a high incidence of viral recurrence following the transplant

20 *A 68-year-old woman with known cirrhosis presents with marked abdominal swelling. Ultrasound examination confirms the clinical suspicion that she has developed ascites.*

Regarding cirrhotic ascites, which of the following statements is true?
a. Ascites only begins to form once the urea and creatinine are elevated
b. The urinary sodium is usually high
c. Plasma renin activity is elevated
d. The associated hyponatraemia should be treated by infusing saline solutions
e. The ascitic fluid characteristically has a high albumin content

21 *A 78-year-old man with known alcohol-related cirrhosis is admitted to hospital with confusion. On examination he has a fetor suggestive of hepatic encephalopathy.*

Which of the following statements is correct?
a. An elevated plasma ammonia is diagnostic of hepatic encephalopathy
b. In a patient with cirrhosis it is rare to find a precipitating cause for encephalopathy so it should just be managed symptomatically
c. Insertion of a TIPS is an effective treatment for hepatic encephalopathy
d. The absence of an asterixis excludes hepatic encephalopathy
e. Hepatic encephalopathy may be precipitated by diuretics

22 *A 54-year-old woman presents with a long history of pruritus and lethargy. Blood tests reveal that her alkaline phosphatase is elevated at 484 iU/L, her bilirubin is 54 μmol/L and ALT is normal. On examination she is slightly pigmented with bilateral xanthelasma.*

Which one of the following statements is true?
a. She should be started on steroids for presumed autoimmune hepatitis
b. Antimitochondrial antibodies are likely to be positive
c. A liver biopsy is a mandatory investigation

d. Her liver disease is an adequate explanation for her elevated alkaline phosphatase
e. She should have cholesterol-lowering therapy even if her blood cholesterol is in the normal range

23 *A 38-year-old man with history of alcohol excess is admitted to hospital following a haematemesis. At endoscopy he is found to have large oesophageal varices that are banded.*

Regarding the management of patients with bleeding oesophageal varices, which of the following statements is true?
a. Emergency surgery is often performed if it is not possible to control the bleeding endoscopically
b. If bleeding is controlled at the initial endoscopy no further endoscopic management is required
c. Balloon tamponade is a low risk procedure and a Sengstaken–Blakemore tube should be inserted in all cases of major bleeding
d. Terlipressin administration does not affect mortality from variceal bleeding
e. Insertion of a TIPS decompresses the varices and can control bleeding

24 *A 57-year-old man presents with an elevated ALT of 157 iU/L. His medical history includes emphysema and osteoarthritis. He has a normal body mass index. He drinks 10 units of alcohol a week and has a 20 pack year smoking history. His brother died of liver cancer aged 62 years. A liver ultrasound demonstrates a cirrhotic looking liver but no evidence of portal hypertension.*

What is the most likely diagnosis?
a. Cystic fibrosis
b. Alpha-1 antitrypsin deficiency
c. Hepatic hydrothorax
d. Haemochromatosis
e. Hepatopulmonary syndrome

25 *A 45-year-old woman presents with diarrhoea and facial flushing. She has no other medical history. On examination she is well and apyrexial but has hepatomegaly. A CT scan reveals multiple arterial-enhancing lesions within her liver.*

What is the most likely diagnosis?
a. Breast carcinoma with metastatic disease
b. Liver abscesses
c. Carcinoid syndrome
d. Colorectal liver metastases
e. Multiple hepatic adenomas

26 *A 57-year-old woman with jaundice and coagulopathy is assessed for liver transplantation.*

Which one of the following are contraindications to liver transplantation?
a. Cholangiocarcinoma
b. Hepatocellular carcinoma
c. HIV infection
d. Hepatitis C virus infection
e. Paracetamol-induced liver failure

27 *A 58-year-old woman presents to her doctor having developed jaundice. She is normally well apart from having had an infected insect bite 6 weeks previously which was treated with antibiotics. Blood tests reveal bilirubin 128 µmol/L, ALT 214 iU/L and ALP 257 iU/L. Hepatitis A, B and C serology is negative.*

What is the most likely diagnosis?
a. Acute autoimmune hepatitis
b. Budd–Chiari syndrome
c. Drug-induced liver injury
d. CMV hepatitis
e. Primary biliary cirrhosis

28 *A 48-year-old man is referred to the hepatology department as he has an elevated ALT of 179 iU/L. He is well in himself but has a body mass index of 37 kg/m². He drinks 10 units of alcohol a week. He has a family history of diabetes and ischaemic heart disease with his father dying of a myocardial infarction aged 55 years. Blood tests looking for evidence of chronic liver disease are negative and he undergoes a liver biopsy which shows simple hepatic steatosis.*

Which one of the following statements is true?
a. As there is no inflammation or fibrosis in his liver he is not at risk of future liver disease and he should be reassured and discharged
b. There is no specific treatment to recommend
c. Alcohol-induced steatosis is the most likely diagnosis
d. If he abstains from alcohol his steatosis will resolve and blood tests normalise
e. He should be screened for diabetes and hypercholesterolaemia and treated if appropriate

29 *A 55-year-old woman with a long history of hypothyroidism and vitiligo is referred for investigation as she has been found to have an ALT of 372 iU/L. Her immunoglobulins are elevated and a liver biopsy demonstrates a plasma cell infiltrate within the liver but no fibrosis.*

Which one of the following statements is true?
a. If her liver autoantibodies are negative, autoimmune hepatitis can be excluded
b. There is no fibrosis in the liver so she should be reassured and discharged
c. The appropriate treatment is a short course of oral prednisolone starting at 30 mg a day and tapering down to zero over a fortnight
d. She is likely to require long-term immunosuppression and should therefore start a steroid-sparing agent early
e. She is unlikely to need another liver biopsy

30 *A 37-year-old man with a long history of drinking a bottle of vodka a day is admitted with jaundice and ascites. On examination he is cachectic with a body mass index of 19 kg/m². His bilirubin is 395 μmol/L, ALT 75 iU/L, ALP 101 iU/L, creatinine 110 μmol/L and INR 2.8.*

Which one of the following statements is true?
a. In this setting he is likely to have alcoholic hepatitis and there is no need to seek another diagnosis
b. If the diagnosis is alcoholic hepatitis he has a 50% chance of dying during this admission to hospital
c. If the diagnosis is alcoholic hepatitis there is no specific treatment
d. His renal function is normal
e. He requires a low protein diet to reduce the risk of developing encephalopathy

EMQs

1 Jaundice

a. Carcinoma of the head of the pancreas
b. Gilbert's syndrome
c. Common bile duct stones
d. Alcoholic hepatitis
e. Primary sclerosing cholangitis
f. Acute viral hepatitis
g. Paracetamol overdose
h. Decompensated cirrhosis
i. Haemolytic anaemia
j. Primary biliary cirrhosis

For each of the following patients with jaundice select the most likely diagnosis from the list above. Each diagnosis may be chosen once, more than once or not at all.

1. A 25-year-old woman is found at home with confusion, vomiting, jaundice and bilateral subconjunctival haemorrhages. She was completely well 3 days ago but hasn't been to work since. Blood tests reveal bilirubin 248 μmol/L, ALT 4184 iU/L and INR 3.8.
2. A 35-year-old man develops jaundice shortly after a bout of flu. This has happened to him several times in the past. The jaundice always resolves completely within a week and he is well in between episodes. There is a similar history in his mother.
3. A 48-year-old woman presents with jaundice associated with right upper quadrant pain and vomiting. She gives a history of recurrent attacks of right upper quadrant pain, particularly after meals. On examination she is tender in the right upper quadrant but there are no palpable masses.
4. A 65-year-old man presents with gradually increasing jaundice. On examination he has bilateral Dupuytren's contracture, multiple spider naevi and enlargement of the parotid glands. His abdomen is grossly distended with ascites.

5. A 75-year-old woman presents with painless jaundice and weight loss. She was diagnosed with diabetes 3 months previously. Examination of her abdomen reveals a palpable gallbladder.

2 Focal liver lesion

a. Simple cyst
b. Hepatic adenoma
c. Cholangiocarcinoma
d. Haemangioma
e. Hepatocellular carcinoma
f. Metastasis
g. Pyogenic abscess
h. Hydatid cyst
i. Amoebic abscess
j. Focal nodular hyperplasia

For each of the following patients found to have a solitary lesion on liver ultrasound, suggest a diagnosis. Each diagnosis may be chosen once, more than once or not at all.

1. A 58-year-old man presents with cirrhosis secondary to non-alcoholic fatty liver disease and an elevated α-fetoprotein with an arterially enhancing lesion on CT examination of the abdomen.
2. A 67-year-old man presents with malaise, weight loss and intermittent fever 6 weeks after a laparoscopic appendicectomy. He has a 6 cm lesion in the right lobe of the liver that contains multiple small foci of gas.
3. A 34-year-old woman presents with a 12-year history of oral contraceptive use with a focal lesion on liver ultrasound discovered during follow-up for a mildly elevated ALT.
4. A 63-year-old man with a 10-year history of primary sclerosing cholangitis presenting with painless jaundice and pruritus.
5. A 37-year-old man who develops anaphylactic shock during attempted aspiration of a cystic lesion in the liver.

Hepatology: Clinical Cases Uncovered, 1st edition. © Kathryn Nash and Indra Neil Guha. Published 2011 by Blackwell Publishing Ltd.

3 Investigation tests

a. Liver ultrasound
b. ERCP
c. Liver biopsy
d. Chronic liver disease screen
e. MRCP
f. INR
g. CT of the abdomen
h. Ascitic tap
i. Gastroscopy
j. Amylase

For each of the patients described below choose the most appropriate first-line test from the above list. Each answer may be chosen once, more than once or not at all.

1. A 34-year-old woman who has taken a paracetamol dose 2 days previously. She is jaundiced with a bilirubin of 102 μmol/L and her ALT is elevated at 4389 iU/L.
2. A 45-year old-woman presents with jaundice and a 2-year history of recurrent right upper quadrant that develops after meals and lasts for up to 4 hours.
3. An asymptomatic 37-year-old man with a long history of ulcerative colitis who is noted to have an elevated alkaline phosphatase of 259 iU/L. The liver ultrasound appears normal.
4. A 57-year-old woman is noted to have an elevated ALT of 93 iU/L. The ultrasound examination of the liver is normal.
5. A 75-year-old man with a short history of painless jaundice associated with dark urine and pale stools.

4 HBV serology

Patient	HBsAg	HBsAb	Anti-HBc IgM	Anti-HBc IgG	HBeAg	HBeAb	HBV DNA	Anti-δ IgM	ALT
a.	+	−	+	−	+	−	++	−	+++
b.	−	+	−	−	−	−	−	−	Normal
c.	+	−	−	+	+	−	+++	−	Normal
d.	+	−	−	+	−	+	++	−	++
e.	+	−	−	+	−	+	−	+	++
f.	−	+	−	+	−	+	−	−	Normal
g.	+	−	+	−	+	−	+	+	++
h.	−	−	+	−	−	−	−	−	++++
i.	+	−	−	+	+	−	++	−	+++
j.	+	−	−	+	−	+	−	−	Normal

The following patients all have hepatitis B virus. From the table above choose the serology that fits best with each patient described. Each answer may be chosen once, more than once or not at all.

1. A patient presenting with fulminant liver failure secondary to acute hepatitis B infection.
2. A health care worked who has been vaccinated against HBV.
3. A patient with HBV and hepatitis D co-infection.
4. A patient who has recovered from acute hepatitis B virus infection.
5. A healthy chronic carrier in the immunotolerant phase of HBV infection.

5 Jaundice in a neonate

a. Gilbert's syndrome
b. Biliary atresia
c. Alpha-1 antitrypsin deficiency
d. Physiological jaundice
e. Hypothyroidism
f. Congenital cytomegalovirus
g. Crigler–Najjar syndrome type 1
h. Hepatitis B infection
i. Sepsis
j. Hepatitis A infection

6 Abnormal liver function tests

a. Wilson's disease
b. Alpha-1 antitrypsin deficiency
c. Primary biliary cirrhosis
d. Haemochromatosis
e. Primary sclerosing cholangitis
f. Constrictive pericarditis
g. Autoimmune hepatitis
h. Drug-induced liver disease
i. Non-alcoholic fatty liver disease
j. Chronic hepatitis C virus infection

For each of the patients whose history is described below choose the most likely diagnosis from the list above. Each diagnosis may be chosen once, more than once or not at all.

1. A 6-week-old infant presents with stiffness in the limbs and convulsions. He is deeply jaundiced but the colour of his urine and stools are normal. His parents are second cousins and their first child developed a similar problem and died of brain damage at the age of 3 months.
2. A 10-day-old baby has mild jaundice which began on the second day of life. She is otherwise well and her urine and stools are normal in colour. She is breast fed and putting on weight.
3. A 5-week-old baby presents with jaundice. Pregnancy and birth were normal and she was well at birth. Jaundice was first noticed on the second day of life and she has developed dark urine and pale stools.
4. An infant is noted to have jaundice on the day he is born. His mother had had several severe colds through the pregnancy. The baby was born with a low birth weight and was noted to be jaundiced with a small head and a widespread rash.
5. An infant is noted to have jaundice 6 days after delivery. He is unwell, refusing to feed and has a high fever. Examination reveals erythema around his abdomen and a purulent discharge from his umbilical stump.

For each patient described below choose the most likely diagnosis from the list above. Each diagnosis may be chosen once, more than once or not at all.

1. A 67-year-old man is incidentally found to have an elevated ALT of 129 iU/L at his annual diabetic check-up. He has a body mass index of 32 kg/m² and is being treated for hypercholesterolaemia
2. A 13-year-old boy with declining cognitive performance and tremor is found to have an elevated ALT of 192 iU/L.
3. A 35-year-old with haemophilia with lethargy and an ALT of 218 iU/L.
4. A 45-year-old woman with tiredness and pruritus and an ALP of 390 iU/L. She has bilateral xanthelasma and is mildly pigmented.
5. A 58-year-old woman with a previous history of radiotherapy for breast cancer who has developed breathless. On examination she has an elevated jugular venous pressure, hepatomegaly and ascites. Her alkaline phosphatase is elevated at 216 iU/L.

---

7 Ascites

a. Budd–Chiari syndrome

b. Abdominal tuberculosis

c. Cirrhosis

d. Ovarian carcinoma

e. Spontaneous bacterial peritonitis

f. Pancreatitis

g. Congestive cardiac failure

h. Meig's syndrome

i. Metastatic colorectal carcinoma

j. Hypothyroidism

For each of the patients described below choose the most likely cause for ascites from the above list. Each cause may be used one, more than once or not at all.

1. A 67-year-old woman with known cirrhosis presents with confusion. An ascitic tap reveals an albumin of 17 g/L (serum albumin = 25 g/L). The ascitic white cell count is elevated at 500 cells/μL and no organisms are seen; serum CA125 is elevated at 247 iU/mL (normal <37 iU/mL).

2. A 34-year-old Nigerian man presents with fever, night sweats and ascites. An ascitic tap reveals an albumin of 44 g/L (serum albumin = 35 g/L). The ascitic white cell count is elevated with lymphocytes and monocytes seen on microscopy.

3. A 43-year-old man with essential thrombocythaemia presents with sudden onset of abdominal pain. On examination there is painful hepatomegaly and marked ascites. Ascitic fluid examination reveals the fluid to be an exudate with a very high protein content.

4. A 78-year-old man with diarrhoea and weight loss develops abdominal swelling. On examination he has ascites and an enlarged, hard liver. Ascitic fluid is an exudate and has some atypical cells on cytology

5. A 58-year-old man has diabetes and recent onset of ascites. He has a history of high alcohol intake and multiple admissions to hospital for epigastric pain and vomiting. He is thin and has diarrhoea with pale stools. The ascitic fluid has a high protein content.

---

8 Abnormal liver function tests

a. Paracetamol overdose

b. Gilbert's syndrome

c. Primary biliary cirrhosis

d. Pregnancy

e. Non-alcoholic fatty liver disease

f. Biliary atresia

g. Gallstone obstruction of the common bile duct

h. Acute autoimmune hepatitis

i. Focal nodular hyperplasia

j. Cirrhosis

For each patient whose investigation results are shown below choose the most likely diagnosis from the list above. Each diagnosis may be chosen once, more than once or not at all.

1. A 26-year-old woman with stable chronic hepatitis B infection is found to have the following results:

Bilirubin	12 μmol/L	ALT	25 iU/L	ALP	179 iU/L
Albumin	30 g/L	AFP	72 iU/mL		

2. A 31-year-old woman is confused and unwell and has the following blood results:

Bilirubin	157 μmol/L	ALT	8820 iU/L	ALP	215 iU/L
INR	4.2 (with no improvement after the administration of intravenous vitamin K)				

3. A 45-year-old woman with a long history of alcohol intake has the following results:

Bilirubin	15 μmol/L	ALT	36 iU/L	ALP	85 iU/L
INR	1.1	Plt	85 × 10⁹/L		

4. A 42-year-old woman with recurrent episodes of self-limiting jaundice has the following results:

Bilirubin	52 μmol/L	ALT	22 iU/L	ALP	67 iU/L

5. A 42-year-old woman with sudden onset of jaundice has these results:

Bilirubin	178 μmol/L	ALT	82 iU/L	ALP	625 iU/L
INR	2.2 (after giving intravenous vitamin K, the INR falls to 1.0)				

9 Viral hepatitis
a. Hepatitis A virus
b. Hepatitis B virus
c. Hepatitis C virus
d. Hepatitis D virus
e. Hepatitis E virus
f. Cytomegalovirus
g. Ebstein–Barr virus
h. Herpes simplex virus
i. Yellow fever virus
j. Human immunodeficiency virus

10 Causes of cirrhosis
a. Methotrexate
b. Hepatitis C virus
c. Cystic fibrosis
d. Haemochromatosis
e. Hepatitis B virus
f. Primary sclerosing cholangitis
g. Primary biliary cirrhosis
h. Non-alcoholic fatty liver disease
i. Wilson's disease
j. Alpha-1 antitrypsin deficiency

For each patient described below choose the most likely diagnosis from the list above. Each diagnosis may be chosen once, more than once or not at all.

1. A pregnant woman who died of acute viral hepatitis shortly after returning from a trip to India.
2. A 35-year-old woman from Zimbabwe who develops acute liver failure following cytotoxic chemotherapy for lymphoma.
3. A 26-year-old man known to have chronic hepatitis B virus presents with jaundice and a sudden deterioration in his liver function.
4. A health care worker who develops an elevated ALT 10 weeks after a needlestick injury from an intravenous drug user in casualty.
5. A man presenting with jaundice and elevated ALT. His homosexual partner has been treated for liver cancer.

Each patient described below has cirrhosis. Choose the most likely cause for cirrhosis from the list above. Each diagnosis may be chosen once, more than once or not at all.

1. A 56-year-old smoker with end-stage emphysema and a family history of cirrhosis.
2. A 67-year-old woman with severe psoriasis who has been managed by the rheumatologists for 20 years.
3. A 19-year-old man with clubbing, a chronic productive cough, steatorrhoea and diabetes.
4. A 55-year -old man with atrial fibrillation, diabetes and impotence.
5. A 48-year-old man with a 10-year history of ulcerative colitis.

SAQs

1 *A 68-year-old man with alcohol-related cirrhosis comes to the accident and emergency department with drowsiness and confusion. On examination he has signs of chronic liver disease and is jaundiced with moderate ascites. His temperature is 38°C and he has a hepatic asterixis.*

a. Why do patients with liver disease get encephalopathy?
b. What factors may precipitate hepatic encephalopathy?
c. Give two important investigations you would undertake in this patient.
d. Briefly outline the management of encephalopathy.

2 *A 37-year-old man presents with a 2-week history of painless jaundice.*

a. How do you classify the causes of jaundice?
b. For each group in (a) describe the classic abnormalities in liver blood tests.
c. For each group in (a) what questions would you ask him?
d. For each group in (a) what signs would you look for on examination?

3 *A 63-year-old woman presents to her GP with abdominal distension. On examination she has palmar erythema, leuconychia and several spider naevi. Abdominal examination reveals fullness in the flanks with shifting dullness. Investigation reveals a serum-ascites albumin gradient (SAAG) of 15 g/L.*

a. What is the SAAG?
b. Give at least three causes of ascites with a low SAAG (<11 g/L) and three causes of ascites with a high SAAG (>11 g/L).
c. Why do patients with liver disease get ascites?
e. Outline the management of ascites in a patient with liver disease.

4 *A 47-year-old man with a long history of alcohol excess presents to casualty with haematemesis and melaena. On examination he is pale; his pulse is 110 beats per minute and BP is 85/60 mmHg. He is jaundiced with signs of chronic liver disease and ascites.*

a. Give a differential diagnosis for the most likely causes of gastrointestinal bleeding in this patient.
b. Briefly outline the immediate management steps.
c. What endoscopic treatments are available for treating acute variceal haemorrhage?
d. What other non-endoscopic treatments are important in this patient?

Hepatology: Clinical Cases Uncovered, 1st edition. © Kathryn Nash and Indra Neil Guha. Published 2011 by Blackwell Publishing Ltd.

PART 3: SELF-ASSESSMENT

5 *A 41-year-old woman is referred to the hepatology clinic as her brother has been diagnosed with genetic haemochromatosis. Her general practitioner has checked her serum ferritin, which is elevated at 479 ng/mL. She has a BMI of 34, her ALT is elevated at 210 iU/L and a liver ultrasound suggests a fatty liver.*

a. What is genetic haemochromatosis?
b. How likely is she to have this disorder?
c. What tests would you do?
d. What organs or tissues are affected by genetic haemochromatosis?

6 *A 58-year-old man is admitted with jaundice. His blood tests are as follows:*
Bilirubin   93 μmol/L (0–20 μmol/L)
ALT   103 iU/L (10–40 iU/L)
ALP   792 iU/L (35–105 iU/L)

A liver ultrasound is performed, which demonstrates a dilated intrahepatic and extrahepatic biliary system.
a. Classify the causes of biliary obstruction.
b. For each group in (a) give a differential diagnosis for biliary obstruction in this case.
c. What investigations would you consider doing next?
d. What methods are available for relieving biliary obstruction?

7 *A 34-year-old woman presents with jaundice and right upper quadrant discomfort after a 2-week history of feeling unwell with nausea, anorexia, myalgia and lethargy. Blood tests are as follows:*
Bilirubin   165 μmol/L
ALT   1926 iU/L
ALP   192 iU/L

a. What pattern of abnormality is seen in her liver function tests?
b. Give a differential diagnosis.
c. What test must be performed urgently?
d. What other investigations would you do?

8 *A 64-year-old woman is investigated for right upper quadrant pain. A liver ultrasound demonstrates three lesions within the liver.*

a. How would you classify lesions within the liver?
b. Give a differential diagnosis using the classification in (a).
c. What questions would you ask?
d. What investigations should be performed?

9 *A 53-year-old man with a long history of excess alcohol use is found to have abnormal liver function tests with an ALT of 138 iU/L.*

a. What pathological effects does alcohol have on the liver?
b. List at least six effects of alcohol on organs or systems other than the liver.
c. What are the complications of acute alcoholic hepatitis?
d. Briefly outline the management of a patient with acute alcoholic hepatitis.

10 *A 65-year-old man is found to have an elevated ALT at a diabetic annual review. Ultrasound examination demonstrates an irregular, nodular liver characteristic of cirrhosis.*

a. What is cirrhosis?
b. Give at least six causes of cirrhosis.
c. What are the complications of cirrhosis?

MCQ answers

1. e: The history of recurrent post-prandial right upper quadrant pain is very suggestive of gallstones. The most likely diagnosis is therefore gallstone obstruction of the common bile duct resulting in jaundice. In suspected biliary obstruction the most appropriate radiological test is an abdominal ultrasound to look for biliary duct dilatation. Carcinoma of the head of the pancreas typically causes painless jaundice and would be uncommon in this age group. In gallstone disease, chronic inflammation usually results in a shrunken fibrotic gallbladder; gallbladder distension is more likely in obstructive jaundice not due to stones. Urobilinogen is colourless; dark urine occurs due to excess conjugated bilirubin passing into the urine. In biliary obstruction there is impaired absorption of the fat-soluble vitamins A, D, E and K. The absence of vitamin K reduces hepatic production of clotting factors resulting in prolongation of the prothrombin time.

2. d: Many infants develop transient jaundice after birth due to the immaturity of the bilirubin conjugating system. It develops on the second day and persists for 2–3 weeks. It is more common in breast fed babies. The colour of the urine and stool are normal. Biliary atresia causes biliary obstruction, the urine turns dark and the stools are pale. Babies with neonatal CMV infection are often unwell and failing to thrive and may have congenital abnormalities. Crigler–Najjar syndrome causes severe hyperbilirubinaemia and untreated can lead to the neurological syndrome of kernicterus. Hypothyroidism is rare but should be excluded if the jaundice persists beyond 3 weeks.

3. c: After assessing that he has a safe airway, the first priority of management is fluid resuscitation. He should be given intravenous fluids, including blood and clotting products if appropriate, prior to undergoing endoscopy. The management of variceal haemorrhage has improved considerably in the past decade and his risk of dying on this admission to hospital is 15–20%. There is evidence that early administration of broad spectrum antibiotics results in a reduction in infection rates, reduced re-bleeding and an improved mortality. Terlipressin causes *vasoconstriction* of the splanchnic circulation, reducing flow and pressure in the portal venous system. The best endoscopic treatment is variceal band ligation. If endoscopic injection is required then a sclerosant agent such as ethanolamine is used rather than adrenaline.

4. c: His bilirubin is elevated but liver enzymes are normal. This suggests that there is no damage to the liver and diagnoses such as viral hepatitis, cirrhosis and drug damage are unlikely. Gilbert's syndrome results from an impairment of bilirubin conjugation, due to a deficiency of transcription of the gene encoding the conjugating enzyme. In illness this transcription is further impaired and the patient may become frankly jaundiced. The rest of the liver function tests are normal. Gilbert's syndrome is suggested by demonstrating that the elevated bilirubin is unconjugated and excluding haemolysis (normal reticulocyte count, serum lactate dehydrogenase, haptoglobin). Jaundice associated with hepatitis A, EBV infection, cirrhosis and paracetamol overdose would cause a conjugated hyperbilirubinaemia and there would usually be other abnormalities of liver function.

5. c: She is in the immunotolerant phase of chronic hepatitis B infection characterised by HBeAg positivity and high levels of HBV DNA in the blood. There are high levels of viral replication but

Hepatology: Clinical Cases Uncovered, 1st edition. © Kathryn Nash and Indra Neil Guha. Published 2011 by Blackwell Publishing Ltd.

PART 3: SELF-ASSESSMENT

as her immune system is not reacting to this there is minimal liver damage and the liver blood tests are normal. In this situation she does not require antiviral treatment but needs to be monitored in the clinic as she remains at risk of developing immune reactivation and a flare of hepatitis. With HBeAg positivity and high levels of HBV DNA she is highly infectious to others. She mostly likely acquired the infection in Pakistan where the prevalence of HBV is high. Infections acquired in this area of the world are most commonly transmitted by the vertical route or early childhood contact. Anti-HB-core IgM antibody is associated with acute infection; as she is a chronic carrier of HBV the IgM anti-HBc will be negative.

6. e: Focal lesions of the liver are an extremely common incidental finding on imaging and are not usually the cause of the symptom for which the scan was organised. In this case the gallstones are much more likely to be the cause of her pain. Most lesions detected incidentally are benign. The correct management is to review the images with an experienced hepatobiliary radiologist to decide whether further imaging is required to fully characterise the lesion. This will usually allow the patient to be reassured and discharged. It is very rare that lesions need to be biopsied. The oral contraceptive pill is associated with development of some liver lesions (e.g. adenoma) and may have to be stopped.

7. b: Alpha-fetoprotein (AFP) may be elevated in HCC and can be a useful screening test for this disorder. However. many HCCs are associated with a normal AFP and an elevated AFP can be associated with conditions without HCC (e.g. testicular tumours, chronic viral hepatitis, liver regeneration). HCCs take their blood supply from the hepatic arterial circulation, therefore characteristic CT features are arterial enhancement of the lesion followed by washout in the portal venous phase. Ultrasound is frequently able to demonstrate an HCC as a hypoechoic lesion even on the background of a nodular liver. Further characterisation with a CT or MRI is recommended. In some situations it is necessary to confirm the suspicion of HCC by undertaking a liver biopsy; however, in many cases the imaging appearances are strongly suggestive and liver biopsy is not required. HCC is rarely symptomatic in the early phases, therefore

high-risk patients (particularly those with cirrhosis) should be entered into a surveillance programme and undergo ultrasound imaging ± AFP estimation every 6 months.

8. a: Primary sclerosing cholangitis is associated with ulcerative colitis, particularly in men. It affects intra- and extrahepatic bile ducts and characteristically produces an elevation in alkaline phosphatase. Primary biliary cirrhosis tends to affect middle-aged women and there is no association with inflammatory bowel disease. Autoimmune hepatitis is associated with ulcerative colitis but is more likely to produce a rise in transaminases. Azathioprine hepatotoxicity and metastatic disease are possible but less likely diagnoses.

9. b: The very high ALT suggests inflammation of the hepatic parenchyma, a hepatitis. Acute viral hepatitis is the most likely cause and characteristically has a viral prodrome before the onset of jaundice, as in this case. Wilson's disease is a possible diagnosis but it is exceptionally rare and therefore less likely to be the cause. Biliary obstruction from gallstones is typically more painful and associated with more marked elevations in alkaline phosphatase rather than ALT. Gilbert's syndrome gives an isolated hyperbilirubinaemia, other liver enzymes are normal. In alcoholic hepatitis the ALT is rarely elevated to more than 200–300 iU/L.

10. e: Acute hepatic ischaemia may be asymptomatic. It can be associated with large increases in transaminases and sometimes impaired synthetic function. The liver is relatively protected from ischaemic insults due to its dual blood supply; however the combination of hepatic congestion and hypotension can provoke hepatic ischaemia, as in this case. Viral hepatitis should always be excluded in any patient presenting with acute hepatitis, but there would often be a history of viral prodrome. The time course of his deterioration is too rapid for a drug-induced liver injury, which often takes several weeks to develop. If Budd–Chiari syndrome presents acutely there is usually abdominal pain and ascites. Haemochromatosis does not usually present with acute symptoms.

11. d: N-acetyl cysteine should be given as determined by the paracetamol levels in the blood drawn at a known time following the overdose. Patients on

enzyme-inducing drugs (e.g. anticonvulsants) and alcoholics metabolise paracetamol to its toxic metabolite more rapidly and should be treated at lower serum levels of paracetamol. Guidelines for treatment are available in all emergency departments. Renal failure is relatively common following a significant paracetamol overdose and occurs due to a direct renal tubular injury by paracetamol. The plasma ALT frequently rises into the thousands but has little bearing on the outcome, the important test is whether the liver retains synthetic function, as assessed by the blood coagulation. For that reason, derangement in coagulation should not be corrected unless there is life-threatening bleeding.

12. a: Intrahepatic cholestasis of pregnancy usually presents in the third trimester with pruritus. Liver function tests are frequently abnormal but jaundice is uncommon. Patients usually have elevated bile acids. The condition resolves following delivery but often recurs in subsequent pregnancies. Acute fatty liver of pregnancy is a more serious condition associated with jaundice, vomiting and abdominal pain. Patients may progress to acute liver failure. The HELLP syndrome (haemolysis, elevated liver enzymes and low platelet count) is a severe form of pre-eclampsia that may result in disseminated intravascular coagulation. It resolves after delivery. If there is derangement of liver function tests in pregnancy other causes must always be excluded but it is rare for hepatitis C and PBC to present acutely.

13. c: Haemochromatosis can cause abnormal liver function tests secondary to iron deposition in the liver. Excess iron can also be deposited in other organs including the pancreas (diabetes), heart (arrhythmia and cardiac failure), skin (pigmentation) and endocrine organs. Arthritis can occur as a result of calcium pyrophosphate deposition in joints. Drug-induced liver disease is unlikely as the medications this patient is taking are not usually hepatotoxic. Wilson's disease presents in young people, usually under the age of 40 years. Congestive cardiac failure is more likely to result in an elevated alkaline phosphatase than ALT. Alpha-1 antitrypsin deficiency is not associated with cardiac, endocrine or joint problems.

14. d: A low caeruloplasmin suggests the disease but levels can be low in acute liver failure of any cause or in heterozygote carriers of the condition. Kayser–Fleischer rings are suggestive of neurological Wilson's disease but they are not specific and can be present in chronic cholestasis of other causes. They are absent in up to 50% of patients presenting with hepatological involvement. Liver disease normally presents in children, and presentation after the age of 40 is extremely rare. Penicillamine is the most commonly used drug to treat Wilson's disease. Neurological symptoms may get worse on commencing treatment.

15. c: Acute hepatic vein occlusion (Budd–Chiari syndrome) results in obstruction to the outflow of blood from the liver causing hepatic congestion, which presents as painful hepatomegaly and ascites. Up to half of cases of Budd–Chiari have an underlying myeloproliferative disorder such as polycythaemia rubra vera as a cause of the hypercoagulable state. Hepatic venous outflow obstruction should always be considered in a patient presenting with painful hepatomegaly and ascites. All the other causes are possible diagnoses but the pain is not typically as severe a feature.

16. d: The major differential diagnosis for his jaundice is progressive PSC with benign structuring of his bile ducts or the development of a cholangiocarcinoma. It can be very difficult to determine this. A MRCP is useful to look at the anatomy of the bile ducts and the nature of the stricturing; benign and malignant strictures may have characteristic features. Cross-sectional imaging (CT or MRI) will be helpful to look for the presence of a mass lesion. CA19.9 can be elevated in biliary obstruction of any cause and is not specific for a cholangiocarcinoma in this setting. Cholangiocarcinoma may be poorly visualised on ultrasound and the lack of a mass lesion is not reassuring. Cholangiocarcinoma is a contraindication for liver transplantation due to the very high risk of the tumour recurring.

17. a: Sexual transmission of HCV in heterosexual monogamous relationships is considered to be extremely rare and no specific precautions are recommended. Sexual practice involving a high risk of trauma to the anogenital mucosa, however, has been associated with an increased risk of transmitting the virus. It is not just sharing needles that puts intravenous drug users at risk of transmitting the virus; transmission has also been

associated with sharing equipment for preparing the drugs (e.g. cookers, spoons, water, etc.). HCV may be associated with vertical transmission but the risk is low, about the order of 6%. It is rarely passed on by breast feeding and patients should not be discouraged from doing this. A needlestick injury from an HCV-positive person is associated with approximately a 3% risk of transmitting the virus (with hepatitis B virus it is approximately 30% and with HIV it is 0.3%).

18. b: The main contraindications to percutaneous liver biopsy include: coagulopathy (INR >1.4, platelet count <60 × 10⁹/L), the presence of significant ascites (as bleeding into the ascites could occur), a dilated biliary system (bleeding could result in haemobilia), infection in the biliary system (risk of disseminating sepsis) and an uncooperative patient. In patients with coagulopathy or ascites, liver biopsy may be performed safely via the transjugular route. The risk of mortality following a liver biopsy is *0.05–0.001%*. Complex cystic lesions should be evaluated with great caution before considering biopsy and negative hydatid serology should be confirmed prior to biopsy since biopsy of a hydatid cyst can be associated with severe anaphylactic shock.

19. d: The current treatment for HCV is a combination of pegylated interferon and ribavirin; it is associated with sustained viral eradication in about 50% of patients (70–80% in patients with viral genotype 2 or 3 and 35–40% in patients with other genotypes). Most people who acquire HCV infection are asymptomatic; acute hepatitis and jaundice is rare. The majority of people exposed to the virus (approximately 85%) progress to chronic infection and are at risk of sustaining liver damage. Not all patients develop progressive liver disease however; the incidence of cirrhosis is approximately 10% at 10 years after infection and 20% at 20 years, and plateaus thereafter. If a patient clears the virus (either naturally or following antiviral therapy), HCV RNA is lost from the serum but HCV antibodies normally remain, therefore these individuals will retain a positive HCV antibody test. Cirrhosis secondary to chronic HCV infection is the leading indication for liver transplantation in most centres. Viral recurrence is nearly universal, however, and associated with more rapid liver injury.

20. c: In cirrhosis there is an alteration in splanchnic haemodynamics resulting in vasodilatation with pooling of blood in the splanchnic system. Consequently, the systemic circulation is underfilled resulting in renal hypoperfusion. This in turn activates the rennin–angiotensin–aldosterone system resulting in an elevation of plasma renin activity. The high aldosterone leads to avid sodium and water retention, thus urinary sodium levels are often low. Hyponatraemia often occurs but, as total body sodium is already elevated, it is not helped by infusion of saline; treatment is aimed at restricting water intake. Ascites usually begins to form before urea and creatinine become deranged, once they do it may signify the hepatorenal syndrome, a condition associated with a high mortality. Cirrhotic ascites is a transudate and the albumin content is usually low unless it is complicated, e.g. by infection or malignancy.

21. e: Diuretics may precipitate encephalopathy by causing dehydration and electrolyte disturbances, particularly derangement of sodium and potassium. There are many precipitants for encephalopathy and these should be actively sought and reversed if possible (e.g. infection, bleeding, drug toxicity, etc.). Blood ammonia levels may be elevated in hepatic encephalopathy but there are other causes, including urea cycle disorders and other metabolic disorders. Insertion of a TIPS may precipitate or worsen existing hepatic encephalopathy as it allows a portion of the portal venous blood supply to bypass the liver, enter the systemic circulation and reach the brain. It also causes an element of hepatic ischaemia, reducing the ability of the liver to perform its metabolic functions. A hepatic asterixis or flap may be present in encephalopathy but it is often absent in the early phases and later when the patient becomes drowsy. It is not diagnostic of the disorder and may be seen in other conditions such as carbon dioxide retention.

22. b: This woman has a classic presentation of primary biliary cirrhosis in a relatively advanced form. Antimitochondrial antibodies (AMAs) are positive in approximately 95% of cases. If the biochemical and clinical features of the presentation are typical and AMAs are positive a liver biopsy is not necessary to make the diagnosis. Steroids are not used to treat PBC as they are

associated with worsening of the osteoporosis associated with this disorder. Whilst her liver disease is likely to be a key cause of the elevated alkaline phosphatase, her cholestasis also puts her at risk of deficiency of fat-soluble vitamins (A, D, E and K). Vitamin D deficiency can lead to osteomalacia and an elevation of the bone isoenzyme of alkaline phosphatase. Hypercholesterolaemia and the development of xanthelasmata are common in PBC but there is no clear evidence that it is associated with an increase in cardiovascular morbidity and treatment of patients with normal levels of cholesterol is not required.

23. e: A TIPS creates a communication between branches of the intrahepatic portal and hepatic veins forming a portosystemic shunt. This provides a low resistance route for blood to flow through the liver, reducing the portal venous hypertension and decompressing the varices, which usually arrests bleeding. It is often employed when endoscopic methods have failed to control the bleeding. The advent of TIPS has almost completely replaced emergency shunt surgery in the management of these patients. Occasionally, patients require balloon tamponade of bleeding varices to allow safe transfer for emergency endoscopy or TIPS. This procedure is associated with a high risk of complications, however, and should only be performed if bleeding cannot be controlled by another means. Patients who have successful endoscopic therapy should have repeat endoscopy and banding at 1–2-week intervals until the varices have been eradicated. Terlipressin reduces bleeding and has also been shown to reduce the mortality associated with variceal bleeding.

24. b: Alpha-1 antitrypsin is an inherited disorder resulting in accumulation of α_1-antitrypsin globules within hepatocytes, which can eventually lead to cirrhosis. Smokers in particular are at risk of lung injury due to unopposed action of proteolytic enzymes in the lungs. Cystic fibrosis can cause respiratory symptoms and cirrhosis but usually presents in childhood or as a young adult. Haemochromatosis is an inherited disorder that can cause cirrhosis and may also be associated with arthritis but not respiratory involvement. Hepatic hydrothorax occurs when ascites tracks into the pleural space. Features of portal hypertension

would usually be evident. Porto-pulmonary hypertension is also a complication of portal hypertension associated with the development of pulmonary arterial hypertension, which produces breathlessness.

25. c: The history is typical of the carcinoid syndrome. Symptoms occur because 5-HT produced from the liver lesions is able to access the systemic circulation. Breast or colorectal metastases do not usually enhance in the arterial phase on CT scanning and should not produce flushing. Abscesses produce arterially enhancing lesions in the liver but the patient is usually quite unwell with a fever. Hepatic adenomas should not have systemic symptoms.

26. a: Cholangiocarcinoma is currently an absolute contraindication to liver transplantation as it has an extremely high incidence of recurrence after the transplant. In contrast, small hepatocellular carcinomas are a very good indication for liver transplantation and if patients are carefully selected the incidence of recurrence after transplantation is low. Patients have to fit criteria regarding the size and number of lesions and there must not be any evidence of spread outside the liver or invasion of the major vascular structures. HIV infection is not an absolute contraindication to transplantation, although infection that is not amenable to antiretroviral therapy or a diagnosis of AIDS is. Cirrhosis caused by HCV infection is the commonest indication for liver transplantation in the Western world. Transplantation is often indicated for paracetamol-induced liver failure in patients who meet defined criteria that predict a very low chance of spontaneous recovery.

27. c: Antibiotics are a common cause of acute liver injury with jaundice. Agents such as flucloxacillin or augmentin can give rise to a cholestatic hepatitis with jaundice. The reaction may occur a few weeks after stopping the drug and take several weeks to resolve. Autoimmune hepatitis and CMV hepatitis are possible diagnoses in this woman but are less likely than antibiotic-associated jaundice. Budd–Chiari syndrome typically presents with pain, jaundice and ascites. Primary biliary cirrhosis does not present acutely; patients with this condition usually have a history of lethargy and pruritus for several years and jaundice develops slowly.

28. e: This patient has a high BMI and steatosis in his liver, the most likely diagnosis is therefore non-alcoholic fatty liver disease. Although he has simple steatosis now he is at risk of developing steatohepatitis and fibrosis over the coming years. Furthermore, hepatic steatosis indicates an increased risk of developing the metabolic syndrome with diabetes and premature ischaemic heart disease. He should be advised to lose weight through a diet and exercise regime and other risk factors for steatosis (e.g. diabetes and hyperlipidaemia) should be sought and treated as appropriate. His alcohol intake is a little high and he should be advised to reduce this, but in a man with such an elevated BMI it is unlikely that reducing alcohol alone will improve his liver dysfunction.

29. d: The histological features are suggestive of autoimmune hepatitis and she has other autoimmune disorders making this a likely diagnosis. A proportion of patients do not have positive autoantibodies and this should not put you off the diagnosis if the history and histological features fit. She has active inflammation on her liver biopsy and this has a high chance of progressing and developing fibrosis if left untreated. Treatment is likely to be required long term. Corticosteroids act quickly to control inflammation and should be started as soon as the diagnosis is made. It typically takes over a year to bring about histological remission and steroid-sparing immunosuppression (e.g. azathioprine) is required and should be commenced early on. A repeat liver biopsy is often required to confirm histological remission prior to discontinuing steroids.

30. b: The history and blood results are typical of a diagnosis of acute alcoholic hepatitis; however, other disorders can present in this way or coexist with alcoholic hepatitis. This patient should therefore be fully assessed with blood tests to look for other causes of acute or chronic liver disease and abdominal imaging to look for abnormalities of the hepatic vasculature or focal lesions within the liver. Severe alcoholic hepatitis, as in this case, has a high risk of mortality of the order of 50%. Alcoholic hepatitis should be treated by optimising nutrition and feeding by a nasogastric tube is frequently required. Patients require a high protein diet as they are frequently very malnourished with marked protein loss. His creatinine is at the upper end of normal but as most patients with alcoholic hepatitis have a low muscle mass they should have a lower creatinine. A creatinine near the top of the normal range is therefore often abnormal in these patients and should be taken as an indicator of renal dysfunction.

EMQ answers

1

1. g: Paracetamol overdose. Rapid development of hepatitis with confusion and coagulopathy is highly suggestive of acute liver failure. Bilateral subconjunctival haemorrhage is a feature of paracetamol hepatotoxicity.

2. b: Gilbert's syndrome. Jaundice accompanying a systemic illness is characteristic of Gilbert's syndrome. Jaundice resolves spontaneously and the patient is well in between episodes. It is caused by a reduction in activity of the enzyme responsible for bilirubin conjugation.

3. c: Common bile duct stones. The history of recurrent abdominal pain after meals is typical of biliary colic. A subsequent episode of painful jaundice suggests a gallstone has migrated out of the gallbladder into the common bile duct and is causing obstruction.

4. d: Alcoholic hepatitis. He has evidence of decompensated liver disease (ascites and jaundice). The presence of Dupuytren's contracture, parotid enlargement and florid spider naevi suggest alcohol as the diagnosis.

5. a: Carcinoma of the head of the pancreas. Painless jaundice is typical of pancreatic carcinoma. New-onset diabetes is sometimes a presenting feature as the tumour invades the gland, destroying the islets of Langerhan. A palpable gallbladder in the presence of jaundice is suggestive of pancreatic cancer (Courvoisier's law).

2

1. e: Hepatocellular carcinoma (HCC). HCC occurs most frequently on a background of cirrhosis. Other lesions are uncommon in a cirrhotic liver. A raised α-fetoprotein (AFP) is often observed although some HCCs are associated with a normal AFP. HCC typically takes its blood supply from the hepatic artery and is therefore seen to enhance on the arterial phase of a CT scan.

2. g: Pyogenic abscess. Infection in the gastrointestinal tract can result in pyogenic material entering the portal vein by which it can travel to the liver and establish infection there in the form of single or multiple abscesses. Patients with liver abscesses present unwell with generalised symptoms of infection (e.g. fever, lethargy, weight loss) and may also have right upper quadrant pain.

3. b: Hepatic adenoma. This rare benign tumour is often seen in association with hormone use (e.g. oral contraceptive pill or anabolic steroids). It is frequently asymptomatic and an incidental finding. Occasionally it can present as an emergency with pain and shock due to haemorrhage.

4. c: Cholangiocarcinoma. This malignant tumour of the biliary epithelium frequently develops in patients with longstanding biliary disease, particularly primary sclerosing cholangitis. It may occur in the extrahepatic bile ducts when it usually causes biliary obstruction and jaundice. Intrahepatic cholangiocarcinomas may not cause symptoms until they are large and treatment options are limited.

5. h: Hydatid cyst. These occur during infection with the parasite *Echinococcus*. Eggs are ingested and release small worms that travel in the blood stream to various organs, including the liver, where they can develop into large cysts containing the tapeworm larvae. If this lesion is biopsied, the larvae may be released into the blood stream causing an anaphylactic reaction.

3

1. f: INR. She clearly has marked hepatotoxicity related to her paracetamol overdose as evidenced by her hugely elevated ALT and jaundice. The most important

Hepatology: Clinical Cases Uncovered, 1st edition. © Kathryn Nash and Indra Neil Guha. Published 2011 by Blackwell Publishing Ltd.

question is whether her liver is able to perform synthetic functions and a test of blood coagulation such as the INR is the most appropriate test.

2. a: Liver ultrasound. An ultrasound will look for structural causes for her pain, e.g. gallstones (most likely in this case), focal liver lesions or other abdominal pathology.

3. e: MRCP. An elevated alkaline phosphatase suggests a cholestatic or obstructive problem. In a patient with ulcerative colitis, the fibrotic, structuring biliary disease primary sclerosing cholangitis is likely. This is often well demonstrated on an MRCP examination which is preferred to ERCP as a first-line test as it avoids the risks of pancreatitis, bleeding and infection that can be associated with an ERCP.

4. d: Chronic liver disease screen. There are many causes of an elevated ALT. A full chronic liver disease screen should be checked for patients with deranged liver function tests to exclude a viral, immunological or metabolic cause.

5. a: Liver ultrasound. His history is suggestive of cholestasis. Ultrasound is the first-line investigation; if biliary duct dilatation is present further investigation can be organised to look for an obstructive cause. If there is no duct dilatation it suggests an intrahepatic cholestasis, which will require further evaluation with a detailed drug history, chronic liver disease screen and possibly a liver biopsy.

4

1. h: Fulminant liver failure. Patients presenting with fulminant liver failure secondary to HBV frequently have already cleared the virus from the body. Viral antigens (HBsAg and HBeAg) and HBV DNA are therefore often negative. IgG antibodies have not yet been produced, therefore the only evidence of HBV infection is the IgM anti-HBc antibody. As there is hepatic necrosis ALT is often very high (2000–10 000 iU/L).

2. b: Post-HBV vaccination. HBV vaccine contains only HBsAg, the patient is exposed to no other viral antigens. Therefore, the only antibody produced is anti-HBs, which confers protective immunity.

3. g: Hepatitis B and D co-infection. The patient has IgM antibodies to both HBV core antigen and HDV. The most likely explanation for this is co-infection with the two viruses.

4. f: Clearance of HBV. The presence of anti-HBc indicates that the patient has been exposed to HBV; they have cleared HBsAg and therefore no longer carry the virus. The presence of anti-HBs indicates that they have produced a protective antibody.

5. c: Immunotolerant HBV. In a healthy immunotolerant person large amounts of virus circulate in the body, HBV DNA levels are high but the lack of an immune response results in normal ALT. This occurs prior to HBeAg seroconversion, therefore HBeAg is positive and anti-HBe is negative.

5

1. g: Crigler–Najjar syndrome type 1. This is a rare, autosomal recessive disorder characterised by a total absence of the bilirubin conjugating enzyme. Infants become deeply jaundiced with unconjugated hyperbilirubinaemia. If untreated the unconjugated bilirubin crosses the blood–brain barrier resulting in brain damage (kernicterus) and death.

2. d: Physiological jaundice. Most babies who are breast fed develop mild jaundice in the first 2 weeks of life. It is not present at birth, peaks at 2–5 days and then disappears. It is due to excess destruction of red blood cells and immaturity of the conjugating system in the first days of life. Bilirubin is unconjugated and the urine and stools are normal colour.

3. b: Biliary atresia. A disorder characterised by gradual fibrosis and obliteration of the extra- and intrahepatic biliary ducts. Jaundice begins to develop on the second day and gradually progresses. Bilirubin is conjugated but not excreted into the gastrointestinal tract thus the stools become pale and the urine dark. If infants are operated on early and biliary drainage achieved, excessive liver damage can be avoided, if not the infant develops progressive liver fibrosis and liver failure.

4. f: Congenital CMV infection. This devastating syndrome occurs when a mother develops CMV infection during pregnancy and passes it onto the fetus. Infants are usually of low birth weight and may have abnormalities including microcephaly, retinal damage and brain damage. Pneumonia and hepatitis with jaundice may occur.

5. i: Sepsis from umbilical stump infection. Infection of any site in the neonatal period can impair bilirubin conjugation, resulting in jaundice.

6

1. i: Non-alcoholic fatty liver disease. Fat infiltration of the liver is very common in patients with obesity, particularly those with features of the metabolic syndrome such as diabetes and hypercholesterolaemia.
2. a: Wilson's disease. This is a very rare disorder that presents in young people and can lead to irreversible brain damage or liver damage including acute liver failure or cirrhosis. It should be considered in any young person presenting with liver disease; it would be exceptionally rare for it to present over the age of 40 years.
3. j: Chronic hepatitis C virus infection. Patients who received blood products prior to screening for HCV are at risk of having acquired the virus. Patients with haemophilia were at particular risk as factor VIII was obtained from pooled donated blood making it possible that large number of recipients were infected from a single infected donor.
4. c: Primary biliary cirrhosis. She has a classic presentation of this disorder, which primarily affects middle-aged women and presents with tiredness and features of cholestasis, e.g. pruritus.
5. f: Constrictive pericarditis. She has features of cardiac failure, which in this case is caused by pericardial disease related to her precious radiotherapy. With cardiac failure from any cause, the liver can become congested which results in engorgement with blood, hepatomegaly and ascites.

7

1. e: Spontaneous bacterial peritonitis. Any patient with cirrhosis presenting with deterioration in their clinical condition should be evaluated for the possibility of spontaneous bacterial peritonitis. In this woman the serum–ascitic albumin gradient is 8 g/L indicating that the fluid is an exudate and that a complication such as infection is possible. In this setting, the elevated ascitic white cell count should be assumed to reflect infection. Ascites commonly causes mild elevation of CA125 and does not necessarily indicate ovarian malignancy.

2. b: Abdominal tuberculosis. The ascitic fluid is an exudate and has a high content of cells associated with TB.
3. a: Budd–Chiari syndrome. The development of painful hepatomegaly and ascites should always raise the suspicion of the Budd–Chiari syndrome. This can complicate myeloproliferative disorders and other procoagulant disorders.
4. i: Metastatic colorectal carcinoma. Malignancy is a common cause of ascites. Fluid should always be sent for cytology to look for malignant cells.
5. f: Pancreatitis. Chronic pancreatitis may lead to a pancreatic fistula with a direct communication between the pancreatic duct and the peritoneal cavity. The fluid has a high protein content and an elevated amylase.

8

1. d: Pregnancy. The alkaline phosphatase is raised as it is produced by the placenta; if isoenzymes were checked there would be no elevation in the liver ALP. Albumin is low due to haemodilution that occurs due to the increased plasma volume characteristic of pregnancy. Alpha-fetoprotein is produced by the fetus and elevated levels are seen in maternal blood during pregnancy.
2. a: Paracetamol overdose. She has acute liver failure characterised by coagulopathy. As this is not corrected by vitamin K it is due to a failure of liver synthesis rather than cholestasis. The most common cause of liver failure in the UK is a paracetamol overdose and this is the most likely cause when ALT is elevated to this degree.
3. j: Cirrhosis. Liver blood tests are completely normal but this does not exclude serious liver disease. It is quite common for patients with cirrhosis to have normal liver biochemistry. Other clues need to be sought such as a low platelet count indicating hypersplenism and portal hypertension.
4. b: Gilbert's syndrome. There is an isolated hyperbilirubinaemia making a prehepatic cause of jaundice the most likely. The history is suggestive of the common and benign disorder, Gilbert's syndrome. Providing haemolysis is excluded the patient can be reassured.
5. g: Gallstone obstruction of the common bile duct. The pattern of abnormality in her liver blood tests suggests cholestasis, as would be caused by

obstruction of bile flow. The INR reverses with intravenous vitamin K because this fat-soluble vitamin is not absorbed from the gastrointestinal tract when there is cholestasis.

9

1. e: Hepatitis E virus. Most cases of acute viral hepatitis have a relatively low mortality risk, however acute hepatitis E virus infection produces a particularly devastating illness in pregnant women and the mortality rate is around 20%.
2. b: Hepatitis B virus. Chronic hepatitis B virus infection is very common in African countries such as Zimbabwe. Chronic carriers are often well but if the immune system is disturbed, such as with chemotherapy, it can lead to an aggressive hepatitis that can lead to liver failure and be fatal.
3. d: Hepatitis D virus. There are many causes of a patient with hepatitis B virus deteriorating but superadded hepatitis D virus infection should always be considered.
4. c: Hepatitis C virus. Intravenous drug users are at risk of having chronic hepatitis B and C viruses. A health care worker is probably vaccinated against hepatitis B virus, therefore it is more likely that they have acquired hepatitis C virus.
5. b: Hepatitis B virus. Hepatitis B is spread by sexual contact, both heterosexual and homosexual. As well as hepatitis and cirrhosis it causes hepatocellular carcinoma.

10

1. j: Alpha-1 antitrypsin deficiency. Deficiency of α_1-antitrypsin predisposes to lung destruction, which presents as emphysema, especially in smokers. Abnormal α_1-antitrypsin globules accumulate in hepatocytes and can lead to the development of fibrosis and cirrhosis.
2. a: Methotrexate. Chronic use of methotrexate for conditions such as psoriasis and rheumatoid arthritis can lead to fibrosis in the liver. If the drug is continued, this can progress to cirrhosis in a minority of cases.
3. c: Cystic fibrosis. Respiratory symptoms predominate in this chronic disorder, however as respiratory treatments have improved patients are living longer and suffer from the effects of thickened secretions on other organs. In the liver this can result in a biliary cirrhosis. Pancreatic involvement can lead to exocrine deficiency (chronic pancreatitis) and endocrine abnormalities (diabetes).
4. d: Haemochromatosis. Iron overload in haemochromatosis affects multiple organ systems including the liver (cirrhosis), pancreas (diabetes), heart (arrhythmias, cardiomyopathy) and endocrine organs (gonadal dysfunction).
5. f: Primary sclerosing cholangitis. This chronic biliary disorder is associated with inflammatory bowel disease.

SAQ answers

1

a. Increased delivery of nitrogenous material to the brain. Many factors are involved, e.g. impaired hepatic metabolism of toxins, nitrogenous material bypassing the liver altogether through portosystemic shunts and overproduction of toxins due to increased risk of infection.

b. Constipation, gastrointestinal bleeding, drugs (e.g. opiates, sedatives), infection, electrolyte disturbances and venous thrombosis.

c. Full septic screen (urine, chest, blood cultures, ascitic tap) and serum electrolytes.

d. Treat any underlying precipitant (e.g. correct electrolyte disturbances, give antibiotics for infection, stop sedative drugs), give laxatives to encourage bowel emptying, and provide general supportive measures for drowsy, confused patients (e.g. ensure airway protection, nutrition, skin care, etc.).

2

a. Prehepatic, hepatic and posthepatic.

b. • Prehepatic: Isolated raised bilirubin (ALT and ALP normal). Bilirubin is unconjugated.
• Hepatic: Rise in ALT is higher than the rise in ALP. Bilirubin is unconjugated and conjugated.
• Posthepatic: Rise in ALP is higher than the rise in ALT. Bilirubin is conjugated.

c. • Prehepatic: Previous history or family history (Gilbert's syndrome); family history of anaemia or splenectomy (haemolysis).
• Hepatic: Alcohol history; viral hepatitis risk (recent travel, blood transfusion, sexual risk, intravenous drug use); drug history (prescribed and over the counter drugs); autoimmune disease history (autoimmune hepatitis, PBC, PSC).

Hepatology: Clinical Cases Uncovered, 1st edition. © Kathryn Nash and Indra Neil Guha. Published 2011 by Blackwell Publishing Ltd.

• Posthepatic: Pain (gallstones); pale stools, dark urine; previous biliary surgery (retained gallstones, biliary stricture); fever/rigor (cholangitis)?
• General: Weight loss (malignancy or advanced liver disease)?

d. • Prehepatic: Anaemia; splenomegaly (haemolysis).
• Hepatic: Systemic features of chronic liver disease (clubbing, spider naevi, palmar erythema, leuconychia, Dupuytren's contracture, bruising, purpura, gynaecomastia); abdomen (ascites, hepatomegaly, splenomegaly, caput medusae).
• Posthepatic: Palpable gallbladder (likely not caused by gallstones); pale stools.

3

a. A calculation made by subtracting the albumin concentration of the ascitic fluid from the albumin concentration of a serum specimen obtained on the same day.

b. • SAAG <11 g/L: High protein-containing ascites, e.g. intra-abdominal malignancy, infection including tuberculosis, pancreatitis, nephrotic syndrome, protein-losing enteropathy.
• SAAG >11 g/L: Low protein-containing ascites, e.g. cirrhosis, congestive cardiac failure, constrictive pericarditis, Budd-Chiari syndrome.

c. • Splanchnic vasodilatation results in relative underfilling of the systemic circulation and renal hypoperfusion. This in turn activates the rennin–angiotensin–aldosterone system resulting in avid salt and water retention.
• Reduced synthesis of plasma proteins, e.g. albumin, results in low plasma oncotic pressure.
• Portal hypertension raises capillary hydrostatic pressure in the splanchnic vascular bed.

d. • Bed rest (if practical) increases renal perfusion and salt and water excretion.
• Low salt diet.

- Diuretics (spironolactone is preferred as it inhibits aldosterone; furosemide may be required in addition).
- Paracentesis with intravenous albumin replacement.
- Transjugular intrahepatic portosystemic shunt in selected cases with good liver function.
- Liver transplantation should be considered in cases of ascites refractory to medical therapy.

4

a. Variceal haemorrhage (oesophageal, gastric), peptic ulcer disease (gastric or duodenal ulceration), mucosal inflammation (oesophagitis, gastritis, duodenitis) and Mallory–Weiss tear.

b. Ensure airway protection, obtain good intravenous access (at least two large bore cannulae) and fluid resuscitation (crystalloid, colloid, blood and clotting factors including platelets). Once the patient is stable proceed to emergency endoscopy.

c. Variceal band ligation (preferred modality of treatment, lower complication rate) and sclerotherapy (injection of ethanolamine, a sclerosant, is effective in controlling bleeding but risks include oesophageal ulceration, perforation and mediastinitis).

d. Administration of vasoactive drug (e.g. terlipressin or octreotide) to reduce splanchnic blood flow and lower the portal blood pressure. Administer intravenous antibiotics to prevent infection and reduce the incidence of rebleeding.

5

a. An inherited disorder of iron metabolism characterised by iron overload with deposition of iron in various tissues of the body.

b. 25% (genetic haemochromatosis is an autosomal recessive disorder). Her serum ferritin is elevated but is not particularly high. This could be because it is caused by an alternative disorder (e.g. non-alcoholic fatty liver disease) or because she is a menstruating female who is protected from iron overload to a certain extent by the monthly blood loss.

c. • Transferrin saturation (useful in patients with a high likelihood of having the disorder, less useful in screening).
• Genetic testing: The majority of cases are homozygous for the C282Y mutation in the *HFE*

gene. A less severe genetic mutation is the H63D mutation which may occasionally be associated with disease in a C282Y/H63D heterozygote. Other genetic causes are described.
• A liver biopsy may be required to assess the degree of hepatic damage and iron overload and to look for alternative causes of her raised liver function tests.

d. Liver (fibrosis, cirrhosis, hepatocellular carcinoma), pancreas (diabetes), skin (bronze pigmentation), heart (arrhythmia, cardiomyopathy, heart failure), joints (arthritis) and endocrine glands (endocrine dysfunction, particularly gonadal failure).

6

a. Intraluminal, mural and extramural.

b. • Intraluminal: Gallstones (common); parasites (rare).
• Mural: Carcinoma (cholangiocarcinoma, ampullary carcinoma); benign biliary stricture (e.g. primary sclerosing cholangitis, biliary inflammation or instrumentation).
• Extramural: Pancreatic carcinoma; duodenal carcinoma; hepatic hilar lymphadenopathy.

c. • MRCP: This demonstrates the anatomy of the biliary system, the site and characteristics of the narrowing and can demonstrate some causes, e.g. gallstones within the bile ducts.
• CT abdomen: This demonstrates the pathology in the surrounding tissues (e.g. pancreas, duodenum). It may demonstrate gallstones but these are often not seen on CT imaging.

d. • ERCP: Endoscopic instrumentation of the biliary system can allow retrieval of stones or dilatation and stenting of the stricture.
Percutaneous transhepatic cholangiogram: Percutaneous puncture of a dilated biliary radical can access the biliary tree and permit drainage of bile as well as dilatation and stenting of strictures.
Surgery: The biliary system may be accessed at surgery where the obstruction can be removed or a loop of bowel can be anastomosed above the obstruction to act as a bypass.

7

a. The striking elevation is in the ALT, which is an enzyme of the hepatocyte and suggests a predominantly hepatitic injury.

b. Acute viral hepatitis (e.g. hepatitis A, B, C or E, CMV, EBV); drug-induced liver injury (consider

prescribed, over the counter or illicit drug use);
acute autoimmune hepatitis; seronegative hepatitis
(liver inflammation without evidence of a viral or
autoimmune cause); Budd–Chiari syndrome;
pregnancy-induced liver failure (usually occurs in
the third trimester); ischaemic hepatitis.

c. INR or prothrombin time to assess whether the liver
is capable of synthetic function.

d. Viral serology (hepatitis B core IgM antibody, IgM
antibodies for hepatitis A, hepatitis E, CMV, EBV,
IgG antibody test for HCV); immunoglobulins; liver
autoantibody screen; caeruloplasmin; liver
ultrasound with Doppler examination of the hepatic
vessels; paracetamol level and other drugs screen.

8

a. Liver lesions can be benign or malignant. Benign
lesions may arise from hepatocytes, biliary
epithelium or other structures. Malignant lesions
can be primary or secondary.

b. • Benign: Hepatocyte origin (focal nodular
hyperplasia, hepatic adenoma); biliary origin (bile
duct adenoma, biliary cyst adenoma); other
(haemangioma, hepatic cyst).
• Malignant: Primary (hepatocellular carcinoma,
cholangiocarcinoma, primary hepatic lymphoma);
secondary (spread from gastrointestinal, lung, breast
or other primary).

c. • Previous cancer elsewhere (breast, lung,
gastrointestinal).
• History suggestive of current cancer elsewhere
(weight loss, respiratory or gastrointestinal
symptoms).
• Risk factors for chronic liver disease: alcohol
intake; risk factors for non-alcoholic fatty liver
disease and the metabolic syndrome (diabetes,
cholesterol, body mass index); viral hepatitis risk
factors; autoimmune disease or inflammatory bowel
disease.

d. • Liver function tests.
• Blood tests to screen for chronic liver disease.
• Tumour markers (α-fetoprotein, CA19.9,
carcinoembryonic antigen, CA125).
• Further imaging after discussion with a radiologist
(e.g. CT scan, MRI scan).

9

a. • Fatty change: Fat is deposited in hepatocytes
mainly in zone 3 of the liver.

• Alcoholic hepatitis: Steatosis is often present.
In addition there are swollen hepatocytes,
hepatocyte necrosis and a neutrophilic infiltrate in
the liver.
• Cirrhosis: Fibrosis surrounds nodules of
regenerating hepatocytes classically in a
micronodular pattern. Steatosis and features of
alcoholic hepatitis may be present.
• Hepatocellular carcinoma: Alcoholic cirrhosis may
be complicated by the development of hepatocellular
carcinoma.

b. • Nervous system: Wernicke–Korsakoff syndrome,
neuropathy, epilepsy.
• Endocrine: Pancreatitis, pancreatic carcinoma,
gonadal dysfunction.
• Cardiovascular: Cardiomyopathy, arrhythmias,
hypertension.
• Gastrointestinal tract: Inflammation, peptic ulcer
disease, carcinoma.
• Muscles: Myopathy.
• Bone: Osteoporosis.
• Bone marrow: Thrombocytopenia, macrocytosis.

c. Liver failure (coagulopathy and bleeding,
encephalopathy), renal failure, sepsis, malnutrition
and death (up to 50% in severe cases).

d. Severe cases need to be admitted to hospital.
Management is largely supportive: optimising
nutrition, including nasogastric feeding if required;
sepsis should be sought and treated promptly;
careful fluid management to detect and treat renal
impairment promptly. Specific treatment with
corticosteroids or pentoxifylline in selected cases.

10

a. Cirrhosis is a response to chronic liver injury. It
affects the whole of the liver, which becomes
replaced by fibrous scar tissue surrounding nodules
of regenerative liver.

b. Alcohol (commonest in the Western world);
hepatitis C virus; hepatitis B virus; non-alcoholic
fatty liver disease; primary biliary cirrhosis;
secondary biliary cirrhosis; primary sclerosing
cholangitis; autoimmune hepatitis;
haemochromatosis; Wilson's disease; α_1-antitrypsin
deficiency; Budd–Chiari syndrome; drugs (e.g.
methotrexate); cystic fibrosis; other metabolic
disorders (e.g. galactosaemia, glycogen storage
disorders).

c. • Liver failure: Jaundice; coagulopathy and bleeding; encephalopathy; increased susceptibility to infection; malnutrition (especially protein catabolism).

• Portal hypertension: Varices and variceal haemorrhage; ascites and functional renal impairment; encephalopathy; splenomegaly and hypersplenism.

• Hepatocellular carcinoma.

Index of cases by diagnosis

Hepatology: Clinical Cases Uncovered, 1st edition. © Kathryn Nash and Indra Neil Guha. Published 2011 by Blackwell Publishing Ltd.

Index

Hepatology: Clinical Cases Uncovered, 1st edition. © Kathryn Nash and Indra Neil Guha. Published 2011 by Blackwell Publishing Ltd.